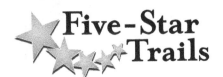

T0152664

Knoxville

0 Spectacular Hikes in the Heart of East Tennessee

2ND EDITION

JOHNNY MOLLOY

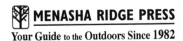

MENASHA RIDGE PRESS
Your Guide to the Outdoors Since 1982

Knoxville

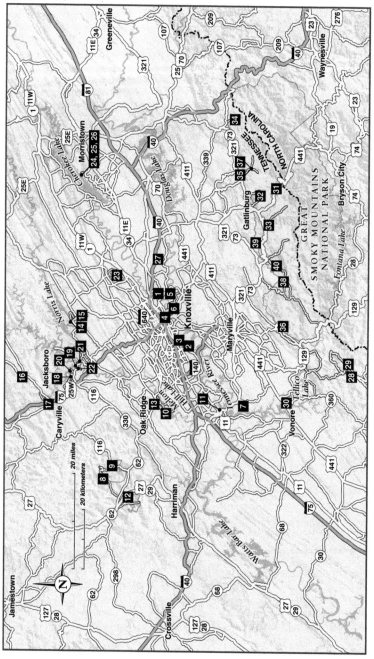

Overview Map Key

Five-Star Trails: Knoxville: 40 Spectacular Hikes in the Heart of East Tennessee
1st edition 2011
2nd edition 2021
Copyright © 2011 and 2021 by Johnny Molloy

Project editor: Kate Johnson
Cover design: Scott McGrew
Text design: Annie Long
Front cover photo: Smoky Mountains National Park in Tennessee. © Sean Pavone/Shutterstock
Back cover photo: Trekking the Cooper Road Trail in autumn. *(See Hike 36, Smoky Mountains: Little Bottoms Loop, page 180.)*
Interior photos: Johnny Molloy, except where noted
Cartography and elevation profiles: Johnny Molloy, Steve Jones, and Scott McGrew
Copy editor: Ritchey Halphen
Indexer: Frances Lennie

Library of Congress Cataloging-in-Publication Data

Names: Molloy, Johnny, 1961- author.
Title: Five-star trails Knoxville : your guide to the area's most beautiful hikes / by Johnny Molloy.
Description: Second edition. | Birmingham, AL : Menasha Ridge Press, 2021.
Identifiers: LCCN 2020048446 (print) | LCCN 2020048447 (ebook) | ISBN 9781634043274 (pbk.)
    | ISBN 9781634043281 (ebook)
Subjects: LCSH: Hiking—Tennessee—Knoxville Region—Guidebooks. | Trails—Tennessee—Knoxville
    Region—Guidebooks. | Knoxville Region (Tenn.)—Guidebooks.
Classification: LCC GV199.42.T22 K666 2021 (print) | LCC GV199.42.T22 (ebook)
    | DDC 796.5109768/85—dc23
LC record available at lccn.loc.gov/2020048446
LC ebook record available at lccn.loc.gov/2020048447

 MENASHA RIDGE PRESS
An imprint of AdventureKEEN
2204 First Ave. S., Ste. 102
Birmingham, AL 35233
menasharidgepress.com
800-678-7006; fax 877-374-9016

Visit menasharidge.com for a complete listing of our books and for ordering information. Contact us at our website, at facebook.com/menasharidge, or at twitter.com/menasharidge with questions or comments. To find out more about who we are and what we're doing, visit blog.menasharidge.com.

All rights reserved
Published by Menasha Ridge Press
Distributed by Publishers Group West
Printed in the United States of America

SAFETY NOTICE Though the author and publisher have made every effort to ensure that the information in this book is accurate at press time, they are not responsible for any loss, damage, injury, or inconvenience that may occur while using this book—you are responsible for your own safety and health on the trail. The fact that a hike is described in this book does not mean that it will be safe for you. Always check local conditions (which can change from day to day), know your own limitations, and consult a map.

For information about trail and other closures due to the coronavirus, check the "Contacts" listings in the hike profiles.

Contents

Dedication

This book is for all of the Tennessee Volunteers. We are blessed with abundant beauty.

 # Acknowledgments

THANKS TO ALL THE PEOPLE who have constructed, maintained, and advocated for trails and hiking in Knoxville and East Tennessee. And thanks to all the people who accompanied me on the trails.

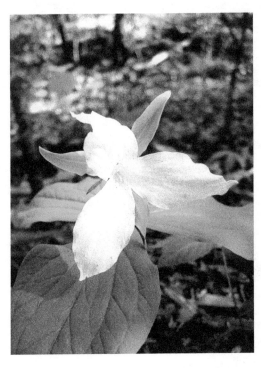

WHITE TRILLIUM GRACES THE TRAILSIDE WOODS AT GALLAHER BEND GREENWAY. *(See Hike 10, page 62.)*

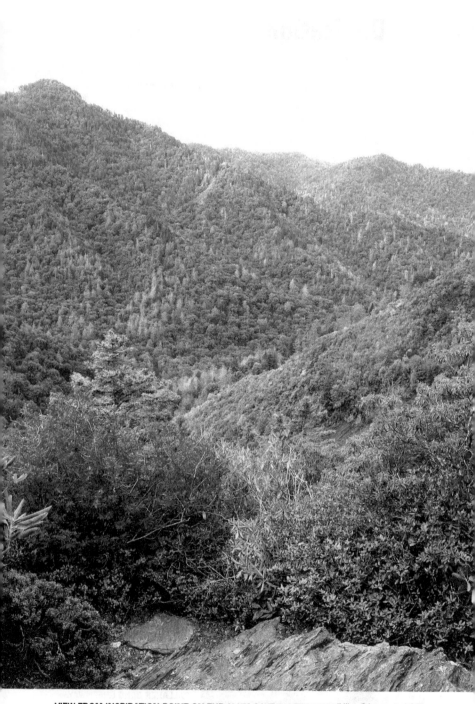

VIEW FROM INSPIRATION POINT ON THE ALUM CAVE BLUFFS HIKE *(Hike 31, page 160)*

Preface

KNOXVILLE IS A HIKER'S TOWN. People like this sport in higher percentages here than in your average city, that's for certain. If somebody is not an avid hiker, they know someone who is.

Talking about trails in Knoxville is as common as conversation about our beloved Tennessee Volunteers sports programs. Knoxville offers an inordinately large number of outdoor stores, far above what you'd think its population could support. Why? The answer is partly geographic and partly cultural.

Geographically speaking, Knoxville couldn't be better situated for terrain and trails on which to trek. The master chain of the Appalachian Range—the Great Smoky Mountains—rises within sight of Knoxville. This span is simply the highest, wildest contiguous plot of rushing streams, rugged ridges, huge trees, colorful wildflowers, and abundant wildlife in the eastern United States. Protected as Great Smoky Mountains National Park, this area has more than 800 miles of hiking trails within its boundaries. Most of the trailheads on the Tennessee side of the park are within an hour's drive of Knoxville, so residents flock to the Smokies. In fact, if you did a street interview and asked people to say the first thing that came to mind upon hearing the word *hike,* the word *Smokies* would likely be chosen most often. The Smokies set the stage for hitting the trail and are the backbone of our hiking community in the heart of East Tennessee.

But there are many more places for a trail treader than that magnificent park. The Cumberland Plateau rises to the west of the Tennessee Valley. The Plateau, as it is known in these parts, offers distinctly different terrain with correspondingly unique hiking experiences. Water-carved gorges slice through this elevated table of land, exposing rock walls and creating rock houses, sheer bluffs, and other geological features that complement the green expanse of the Smokies.

And then there is the ridge-and-valley country north of town, a sort of blending of the Plateau and the high ranges to the east. Here, in places like Norris Dam State Park, narrow hollows are flanked by tightly packed ridges (imagine a rumpled carpet), never particularly high, but nonetheless creating an attractive landscape over which to walk.

No flatland itself, the Tennessee Valley embraces the hilly town of Knoxville. And with citizens interested in hiking, it is only natural that trails and greenways aplenty have been created in the greater metropolitan area. They make going out on a walk not only inviting but also convenient.

So hiking in Knoxville can mean a ramble through the wilds of the Great Smokies, a trip to a geological formation on the Cumberland Plateau, a walk in the deep, dark hollows of the ridge-and-valley country, or a quick escape on a greenway near your house or lodging. It all depends on your mood, company, and desires. It does not necessarily depend on the weather: You can hike year-round in Knoxville. In the heat of summer, you can escape to the high country, and in the chill of winter, you can still enjoy the trails of the Tennessee River Valley.

The variety of hikes in this book reflects the diversity of the region. Day hikes cover routes of multiple lengths, ranging from easy to difficult. Trail configurations include out-and-backs, loops, balloon loops, and even double loops. Destinations vary from downtown Knoxville to the "back of beyond" in the Smokies. The routes also befit a range of athletic prowess and hiking experience.

Simply scan the table of contents, flip randomly through the book, or use the hiking recommendations list on the next page. Find your hike, then get out there and enjoy it. Bring a friend too—enjoying nature in the company of another is a great way to enhance your relationship as well as to escape from smartphones, television, email, internet, and other technology that binds us to the daily grind.

—J. M.

THE WALKER SISTERS' CABIN IN THE SMOKY MOUNTAINS (See Hike 39, page 192.)

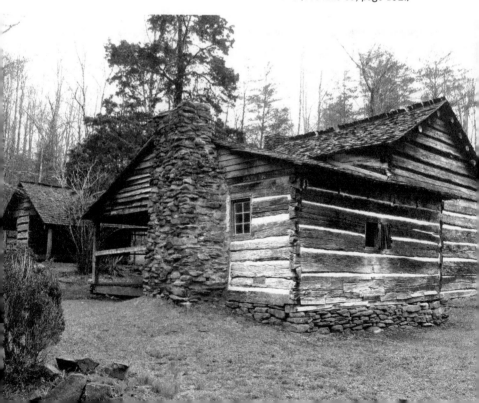

Recommended Hikes

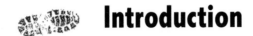 **Introduction**

About This Book

THE SECOND EDITION OF *Five-Star Trails: Knoxville* details 40 great hikes in this city and its immediate region. Often referred to as the heart of East Tennessee, Knoxville is a great jumping-off point for hikers: it's where immediate urban and suburban trails can satiate scenery-hungry residents, while the superlative beauty of the adjacent national and state parks is just a short drive away. All this adds up to a hiker's nirvana.

Greater Knoxville's Geographic Divisions

The hikes in this book are divided into five geographic regions. Altogether, they embrace great destinations such as urban greenways, Great Smoky Mountains National Park, Cherokee National Forest, the Cumberland Plateau, Big Ridge State Park, Frozen Head State Park, and Fort Loudoun State Historic Park.

★ **KNOXVILLE** covers the city core. The hikes here follow mainly along Knoxville's abundant and expanding greenway system. Choose them for a quick escape for daily exercise or to explore nature parks such as Ijams or William Hastie Natural Area.

★ **WEST** encompasses the city of Oak Ridge and public lands west of town, including the Cumberland Plateau. Hike along interpretive trails at the UT Arboretum, climb to the highest point on the Cumberland Plateau at Frozen Head State Park, or try a lakeside greenway.

★ **NORTH** takes in the ridge-and-valley country north of Knoxville and the northward part of the Cumberland Plateau. In this area, you can hike trails around Norris Dam, with views aplenty and wildflowers galore, or take a geologically rewarding trek on the Cumberland Trail, Tennessee's master path.

★ **EAST** stretches from House Mountain State Natural Area to Panther Creek State Park. House Mountain, the highest point in Knox County, has views rivaling those in the Smokies. Panther Creek State Park is unheralded as a hiking destination. Seven Islands State Birding Park will surprise you. The varied topography and combination of land and water will leave you wondering why you haven't been there before.

★ **SOUTH** includes the highest terrain in the region, from the incomparable Smoky Mountains to the remote and unrefined Cherokee National Forest. The Smokies destinations in this guidebook lie within an easy drive from Knoxville and include a medley of pioneer homesteads, panoramic overlooks, and intense waterfalls. The Cherokee trails offer scenery and destinations comparable to those of the Smokies, minus the crowds, and these routes add a primitive component lacking in the more developed pathways of the Smokies.

The trail-laced geographic regions of greater Knoxville create a mosaic of natural splendor that will please even the most discriminating hiker.

How to Use This Guidebook

The following information walks you through this guidebook's organization to make it easy and convenient for you to plan great hikes.

OVERVIEW MAP, OVERVIEW MAP KEY, AND MAP LEGEND

The overview map on page ii shows the primary trailheads for all 40 of the hikes described in this book. The numbers shown on the overview map pair with the map key on the facing page. A legend explaining the map symbols used throughout the book appears on page 17.

TRAIL MAPS

In addition to the overview map, a detailed map of each hike's route appears with its profile. On each of these maps, symbols indicate the trailhead, the complete route, significant features, facilities, and topographic landmarks such as creeks, overlooks, and peaks.

To produce the highly accurate maps in this guidebook, I used a handheld GPS unit to gather data while hiking each route, and then sent that data to Menasha Ridge Press's expert cartographers. Be aware, though, that your GPS device is no substitute for sound, sensible navigation that takes into account the conditions that you observe while hiking. Further, despite the high quality of the maps in this book, the publisher and I think it wise to carry an additional map, such as the ones noted in each hike profile's introductory listing for "Maps," either on paper or on your smartphone.

ELEVATION PROFILE (DIAGRAM)

This diagram represents the rises and falls of the trail as viewed from the side, over the complete distance (in miles) of that trail. On the diagram's vertical axis, or height scale, the number of feet indicated between each tick mark lets you visualize the climb. To avoid making flat hikes look steep and steep hikes appear flat, varying height scales provide an accurate image of each hike's climbing difficulty.

THE HIKE PROFILE

This book contains a concise and informative narrative of each hike from beginning to end. The text will get you from a well-known road or highway to the trailhead, to the twists and turns of the hike route, back to the trailhead, and to notable nearby attractions, if there are any. Each profile opens with the route's star ratings, GPS trailhead coordinates, and other key information. Below is an explanation of the introductory elements that give you a snapshot of each of this book's 40 routes.

STAR RATINGS

The hikes in *Five-Star Trails: Knoxville* were carefully chosen to provide an overall five-star experience, and they represent the diversity of trails found in the region. Each hike was assigned a one- to five-star rating in each of the following categories: scenery, trail condition, suitability for children, level of difficulty, and degree of solitude. It's rare that any trail receives five stars in all five categories; nevertheless, each trail offers excellence in at least one category.

Here's how the star ratings for each of the five categories break down:

FOR SCENERY:

★ ★ ★ ★ ★   Unique, picturesque panoramas
★ ★ ★ ★   Diverse vistas
★ ★ ★   Pleasant views
★ ★   Unchanging landscape
★   Not selected for scenery

FOR TRAIL CONDITION:

★ ★ ★ ★ ★   Consistently well maintained
★ ★ ★ ★   Stable, with no surprises
★ ★ ★   Average terrain to negotiate
★ ★   Inconsistent, with good and poor areas
★   Rocky, overgrown, or often muddy

FOR CHILDREN:

★ ★ ★ ★ ★   Babes in strollers are welcome
★ ★ ★ ★   Fun for anyone past the toddler stage
★ ★ ★   Good for young hikers with proven stamina
★ ★   Not enjoyable for children
★   Not advisable for children

FOR DIFFICULTY:

★ ★ ★ ★ ★   Grueling
★ ★ ★ ★   Strenuous
★ ★ ★   Moderate: won't beat you up— but you'll know you've been hiking
★ ★   Easy, with patches of moderate
★   Good for a relaxing stroll

FOR SOLITUDE:

★ ★ ★ ★ ★   Positively tranquil
★ ★ ★ ★   Spurts of isolation
★ ★ ★   Moderately secluded
★ ★   Crowded on weekends and holidays
★   Steady stream of individuals and/or groups

GPS TRAILHEAD COORDINATES

As noted in "Trail Maps," on page 2, I used a handheld GPS unit to obtain geographic data and sent the information to the publisher's cartographers. In the opener for each hike profile, the coordinates—the intersection of the latitude (north) and longitude (west)—will orient you from the trailhead. In some cases, you can drive within viewing distance of a trailhead. Other hiking routes require a short walk to reach the trailhead from a parking area. Either way, the trailhead coordinates are given from the trail's actual head—its point of origin.

This guidebook expresses GPS coordinates in degree–decimal minute format. For example, the coordinates for Hike 1, Ijams Nature Center Loop (page 20), are as follows:

N35° 57.335' W83° 52.096'

The latitude–longitude grid system is likely quite familiar to you, but here's a refresher, pertinent to visualizing the coordinates:

Imaginary lines of latitude—called *parallels* and approximately 69 miles apart from each other—run horizontally around the globe. The equator is established to be 0°, and each parallel is indicated by degrees from the equator: up to 90°N at the North Pole and down to 90°S at the South Pole.

Imaginary lines of longitude—called *meridians*—run perpendicular to latitude lines. Longitude lines are likewise indicated by degrees. Starting from 0° at the Prime Meridian in Greenwich, England, they continue to the east and west until they meet 180° later at the International Date Line in the Pacific Ocean. At the equator, longitude lines also are approximately 69 miles apart, but that distance narrows as the meridians converge toward the North and South Poles.

To convert GPS coordinates given in degrees, minutes, and seconds to degree–decimal minute format, divide the seconds by 60. For more on GPS technology, see usgs.gov.

DISTANCE & CONFIGURATION

Distance notes the length of the hike round-trip, from start to finish. If the hike description includes options to shorten or extend the hike, those round-trip distances are also included here. **Configuration** defines the type of route—for example, an out-and-back (which takes you in and out the same way), a point-to-point (or one-way route), a figure-eight, or a balloon.

HIKING TIME

Unlike distance, which is a real, measured number, hiking time is an estimate. Every hiker has a different pace. In this guidebook, you can assume the hiking time is based on a pace of about 2 miles per hour (when taking notes and pictures), and that is the standard for most of the hike times. There are some adjustments for steepness, rough terrain, and high elevation. And there is some time built in for a quick breather here and there, but hikers should consider that any prolonged break (such as lunch or swimming) will add to the hike time.

HIGHLIGHTS

Lists features that draw hikers to the trail: mountain or forest views, water features, historical sites, and the like.

ELEVATION

Each hike's key information lists the elevation at the trailhead and another figure for the high or low point on that route. The full hike profile also includes an elevation profile (see page 2).

ACCESS

Trail-access hours are listed here, along with any applicable fees or permits required to hike the trail.

MAPS

Lists recommendations for maps, in addition to those in this guidebook.

FACILITIES

For planning your hike, it's helpful to know what to expect at the trailhead or nearby in terms of restrooms, phones, water, and other niceties.

WHEELCHAIR ACCESS

Listed here is the hike's feasibility for outdoor enthusiasts who use a wheelchair.

COMMENTS

Here you will find assorted nuggets of information, such as whether or not dogs are allowed on the trails. (Note that not every hike has this listing.)

CONTACTS

Listed here are phone numbers, websites, and email addresses for checking trail conditions and gleaning other day-to-day information.

VIEW FROM THE CUMBERLAND TRAIL, TENNESSEE'S MASTER PATH *(See Hike 16, page 88.)*

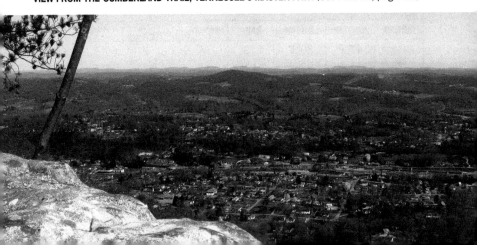

Overview, Route Details, Nearby Attractions, and Directions

These four elements compose the heart of the hike. **Overview** gives you a quick summary of what to expect on that trail; **Route Details** guides you on the hike, from start to finish; and **Nearby Attractions** suggests appealing adjacent sites, such as restaurants, museums, and other trails (not every hike has this listing). **Directions** will get you to the trailhead from a well-known road or highway.

Weather

Each of the four seasons lays its distinct hands on Knoxville. Summer can be fairly hot, but that is when hikers head for the mountains. If you're hiking in Knoxville during summer, I recommend going early in the morning or late in the evening, as thunderstorms can pop up in the afternoons.

Hikers really hit the trails when fall's first northerly fronts sweep cool air across East Tennessee. Mountaintop vistas are best enjoyed during this time. Fall is also the driest of all the seasons here, and crisp mornings give way to warm afternoons.

Winter can bring frigid subfreezing days and chilling rains—and snow in the high country. However, a brisk hiking pace will keep you warm. Each cold month has several days of mild weather.

Spring will be even more variable. A warm day can be followed by a cold one. Extensive spring rains bring regrowth but also keep hikers indoors. Still, any avid trekker will find more good hiking days than they will have time to take on in spring and every other season.

The chart below details Knoxville's monthly averages to give you an idea of what weather to expect. (*Note:* Expect cooler temperatures on the Cumberland Plateau and in the Smokies.)

MONTH	HI TEMP	LO TEMP	RAIN	MONTH	HI TEMP	LO TEMP	RAIN
JAN	47°F	30°F	4.79"	JUL	88°F	68°F	3.97"
FEB	52°F	33°F	3.91"	AUG	87°F	68°F	3.40"
MAR	61°F	40°F	5.04"	SEP	81°F	62°F	3.03"
APR	71°F	61°F	3.52"	OCT	71°F	52°F	3.03"
MAY	78°F	71°F	4.33"	NOV	60°F	41°F	4.10"
JUN	85°F	65°F	4.77"	DEC	50°F	34°F	4.37"

Source: weather.gov

Water

A hiker walking steadily in 90° heat needs about 10 quarts of fluid per 8-hour day. That's 2.5 gallons—10 large (1 quart) water bottles or 16 small (20-ounce) ones. A good rule of thumb is to hydrate before your hike, carry (and drink) 16 ounces of water for every mile you plan to hike, and hydrate again after the hike.

For most people, the pleasures of hiking make the burden of carrying water a relatively minor inconvenience, so pack more water than you think you'll need, even for short hikes. If you don't like drinking tepid water on a hot day, freeze a couple of bottles overnight. It's also a good idea to carry a bottle of sports drink, such as Gatorade; the electrolytes replace essential salts that you sweat out.

If you find yourself tempted to drink found water, proceed with extreme caution. Drinking such water presents inherent risks for thirsty trekkers. *Giardia* parasites contaminate many water sources and can cause giardiasis, an extremely painful gastrointestinal ailment that can last for weeks after onset. For more information, visit the Centers for Disease Control and Prevention website: cdc .gov/parasites/giardia.

In any case, effective treatment is essential before you use any water source found along the trail. Boiling water for 2–3 minutes is always a safe measure for camping, but day hikers can consider iodine tablets, approved chemical mixes, filtration units rated for giardia, and ultraviolet filtration. Some of these methods (for example, filtration with an added carbon filter) remove bad tastes typical in stagnant water, while others add their own taste. As a precaution, carry a means of water purification in case you've underestimated your consumption needs.

Clothing

Weather, unexpected trail conditions, fatigue, extended hiking duration, and wrong turns can individually or collectively turn a great outing into a very uncomfortable one at best—and a life-threatening one at worst. Thus, proper attire plays a key role in staying comfortable and, sometimes, in staying alive. Below are some helpful guidelines.

★ *Choose synthetics, silk, or wool* for maximum comfort in all of your hiking attire— from hats to socks and in between. Cotton is fine if the weather remains dry and stable, but you won't be happy if it gets wet.

★ *Always wear a hat,* or at least tuck one into your day pack or hitch it to your belt. Hats offer all-weather sun and wind protection as well as warmth if it turns cold.

★ *Be ready to layer up or down* as the day progresses and the mercury rises or falls. Today's outdoor wear makes layering easy, with such designs as jackets that convert to vests and zip-off legs.

★ *Wear hiking boots, trail shoes, or sturdy hiking sandals* with toe protection. Flip-flopping on a paved path in an urban botanical garden is one thing, but never hike a trail in open sandals or casual sneakers. Your bones and arches need support, and your toes need protection.

★ *Pair that footwear with good socks.* If you prefer not to sheathe your feet when wearing hiking sandals, tuck the socks into your day pack; you may need them if the weather plummets or if you hit rocky turf and pebbles begin to irritate your feet. And, in an emergency, if you've lost your gloves, you can wear the socks as mittens.

★ *Don't leave rainwear behind,* even if the day dawns clear and sunny. Tuck into your day pack, or tie around your waist, a jacket that is breathable and either water-resistant or waterproof. Investigate different choices at your local outdoor retailer. If you are a frequent hiker, ideally you'll have more than one rainwear weight, material, and style in your closet to protect you in all seasons in your regional climate and hiking microclimates.

Essential Gear

You can buy outdoor vests that have up to 20 pockets shaped and sized to carry everything from toothpicks to binoculars. Or, if you don't aspire to feel like a burro, you can neatly stow all of the following items (listed in alphabetical order, as all are important) in your day pack or backpack.

★ *Extra clothes:* raingear; a change of socks and shirt; and, depending on the season, a warm hat and gloves

★ *Extra food:* trail mix, granola bars, or other high-energy snacks

★ *Flashlight or headlamp* with extra bulb and batteries, for getting back to the trailhead if your hike takes longer than expected

★ *Insect repellent* to ward off ticks and other biting bugs

★ *Maps and a high-quality compass.* Even if you know the terrain from previous hikes, don't leave home without these tools. And, as previously noted, bring maps in addition to those in this guidebook, and consult your maps prior to the hike. If you own a GPS unit, bring that too, but don't rely on it as your sole navigational tool—batteries can die, after all.

    The latest smartphones not only enable you to call for help but also have built-in GPS hardware and software that can help with orientation. (Don't call for help, though, unless you truly need it—remember that your phone's battery can die too.) Smartphones are also valuable for downloading maps to use on the trail, although it's always better to download a map *before* your hike rather than trying to do so on the fly, as coverage can be unreliable in the mountains near Knoxville.

★ *Pocketknife and/or multitool*

★ *Sun protection:* sunglasses with UV tinting, a sunhat with a wide brim, and sunscreen. (*Tip:* Check the expiration date on the tube or bottle.)

★ *Water.* Bring more than you think you'll drink. Depending on your destination, you may want to bring a means of purifying water in case you run out.

★ *Whistle.* It could become your best friend in an emergency.

★ *Windproof matches and/or a lighter,* for real emergencies—please don't start a forest fire.

First Aid Kit

In addition to the preceding items, those that follow may seem daunting to carry along for a day hike. But any paramedic will tell you that the products listed here (again, in alphabetical order, because all are important) are just the basics. The reality of hiking is that you can be out for a week of backpacking and acquire only a mosquito bite. Or you can hike for an hour, slip, and suffer a cut or broken bone. Fortunately, the items listed pack into a very small space. You may also purchase convenient prepackaged kits at your pharmacy or online.

★ Adhesive bandages (such as Band-Aids)

★ Antibiotic ointment (such as Neosporin)

★ Aspirin, acetaminophen (Tylenol), or ibuprofen (Advil)

★ Athletic tape

★ Blister kit (moleskin or an adhesive variety such as Spenco 2nd Skin)

★ Butterfly-closure bandages

★ Diphenhydramine (Benadryl), in case of mild allergic reactions

★ Elastic bandages (such as Ace) or joint wraps (such as Spenco)

★ Epinephrine in a prefilled syringe (EpiPen), typically by prescription only, for people known to have severe allergic reactions

★ Gauze (one roll and a half-dozen 4-by-4-inch pads)

★ Hydrogen peroxide or iodine

Note: Consider your intended terrain and the number of hikers in your party before you exclude any article listed above. A short stroll may not inspire you to carry a complete kit, but anything beyond that warrants precaution. When hiking alone, you should always be prepared for a medical need. And if you're a twosome or a group, one or more people in your party should be equipped with first aid supplies.

General Safety

Here are a few tips to make your hike safer and easier:

★ *Always let someone know where you'll be hiking and how long you expect to be gone.* It's a good idea to give that person a copy of your route, particularly if you're headed into an isolated area. Let them know when you return.

★ *Always sign in and out of any trail registers provided.* Don't hesitate to comment on the trail condition if space is provided; that's your opportunity to alert others to any problems you encounter.

★ *Don't count on a smartphone for your safety.* Reception may be spotty or nonexistent on the trail.

★ *Always carry food and water,* even for a short hike. And, again, bring more water than you think you'll need.

★ *Ask questions.* Public-land employees are on hand to help. It's a lot easier to solicit advice before a problem occurs, and it will help you avoid a mishap away from civilization when it's too late to amend an error.

★ *Stay on designated trails.* Even on the most clearly marked trails, you usually reach a point where you have to stop and consider which direction to head. If you become disoriented, don't panic. As soon as you think you may be off-track, stop, assess your current direction, and then retrace your steps to the point where you went astray. Using a map (paper or digital), a compass, a GPS device or smartphone, and this book, and keeping in mind what you've passed thus far, reorient yourself, and trust your judgment on which way to continue. If you become absolutely unsure of how to continue, return to your vehicle the way you came in. Should you become completely lost and have no idea how to find the trailhead, remaining in place along the trail and waiting for help is most often the best option for adults and always the best option for children.

★ *Always carry a whistle.* It may become a lifesaver if you become lost or hurt.

★ *Be especially careful when crossing streams.* Whether you're fording the stream or crossing on a log, make every step count. If you have any doubt about maintaining your balance on a log, ford the stream instead: use a trekking pole or stout stick for balance, and *face upstream as you cross.* If a stream seems too deep to ford, turn back. Whatever is on the other side isn't worth the risk.

★ *Be careful at overlooks.* While these areas may provide spectacular views, they are potentially hazardous. Stay back from the edge of outcrops, and make absolutely sure of your footing—a misstep can mean a nasty and possibly fatal fall.

★ *Standing dead trees and storm-damaged living trees pose a significant hazard to hikers.* These trees may have loose or broken limbs that could fall at any time. While walking beneath trees, and when choosing a spot to rest or enjoy your snack, *look up.*

★ *Know the symptoms of subnormal body temperature, or hypothermia.* Shivering and forgetfulness are the two most common indicators of this stealthy killer. Hypothermia can occur at any elevation, even in the summer, especially if you're wearing lightweight cotton clothing. If symptoms develop, get to shelter, hot liquids, and dry clothes as soon as possible.

★ *Likewise, know the symptoms of heat exhaustion, or hyperthermia.* Here's how to recognize and handle three types of heat emergencies: **Heat cramps** are painful cramps in the legs and abdomen, accompanied by heavy sweating and feeling faint. Caused by excessive salt loss, heat cramps must be handled by getting to a cool place and sipping water or an electrolyte solution (such as Gatorade). Dizziness, headache, irregular pulse, disorientation, and nausea are all symptoms of **heat exhaustion,** which occurs as blood vessels dilate and attempt to move heat from the inner body to the skin. Find a cool place, drink cool water, and get someone to fan you, which can help cool you off more quickly. **Heatstroke** is a life-threatening condition that can cause convulsions, unconsciousness, or even death. Symptoms include dilated pupils; dry, hot, flushed skin; a rapid pulse; high fever; and abnormal breathing. If you should be sweating and you're not, that's the signature warning sign. If you or a hiking partner is experiencing heatstroke, do whatever you can to cool down and find help.

★ *Most important, take along your brain.* A cool, calculating mind is the single most important asset on the trail. Think before you act. Watch your step. Plan ahead. Avoiding accidents before they happen is the best way to ensure a rewarding and relaxing hike.

Watchwords for Flora & Fauna

Hikers should be aware of the following concerns regarding plants and wildlife, described in alphabetical order.

BLACK BEARS Though attacks by black bears are very rare, they have happened in East Tennessee. The sight or approach of a bear can give anyone a start. If you encounter a bear while hiking, remain calm and never run away. Make loud noises to scare off the bear, and back away slowly. In primitive and remote areas, assume bears are present; in more developed sites, check on the current bear situation prior to hiking. Most encounters are food related, as bears have an exceptional sense of smell and not particularly discriminating tastes. While this is of greater concern to backpackers and campers, on a day hike you may want to enjoy a lunchtime picnic or munch on an energy bar or other snack from time to time, so remain aware and alert.

MOSQUITOES These little naggers are more often found in Knoxville but are also found sparingly in the hillier Plateau and Southern Appalachians. Insect repellent and/or repellent-impregnated clothing are the only simple methods to ward off these pests. In some areas, mosquitoes are known to carry the West Nile virus, so all due caution should be taken to avoid their bites.

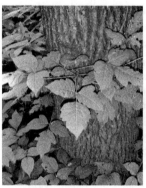

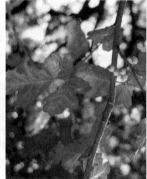

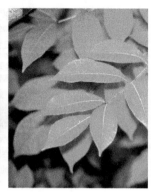

POISON IVY
Tom Watson

POISON OAK
Jane Huber

POISON SUMAC
Norman Tomalin/Alamy

POISON IVY, OAK, AND SUMAC Recognizing and avoiding these plants is the most effective way to prevent the painful, itchy rashes associated with them. Poison ivy occurs as a vine or ground cover, 3 leaflets to a leaf; poison oak occurs as either a vine or a shrub, also with 3 leaflets; and poison sumac flourishes in swampland, each leaf having 7–13 leaflets.

Urushiol, the oil in these plants, is responsible for the rash. Within 14 hours of exposure, raised lines and/or blisters will appear on the affected area, accompanied by a terrible itch. Try to refrain from scratching, because bacteria under your fingernails can cause an infection. Wash and dry the affected area thoroughly with soap and water or a product such as Tecnu; then apply calamine lotion and/or an anti-itch cream. If itching or blistering is severe, seek medical attention. Likewise, make sure to wash any clothes, pets, or hiking gear that may have come in contact with the plant—you could experience a second breakout months after the first if you put on a shirt or a pair of boots that were never properly cleaned.

SNAKES Rattlesnakes, cottonmouths, copperheads, and coral snakes are among the most common venomous snakes in the United States, and hibernation season is typically October–April. In East Tennessee, you will possibly encounter timber rattlers or copperheads, which are most often found along streams or on a sunny spot atop a rock. However, the snakes you are most likely to see while hiking are nonvenomous species and subspecies. The best rule is to leave all snakes alone, give them a wide berth as you hike past, and make sure any hiking companions (including dogs) do the same.

When hiking, stick to well-used trails, and wear over-the-ankle boots and loose-fitting long pants. Don't step or put your hands where you can't see, and avoid wandering around in the dark. Step *onto* logs and rocks, never *over* them, and be especially careful when climbing rocks. Also avoid walking through dense brush. Finally, don't peer into animal burrows, and make sure that dogs don't either.

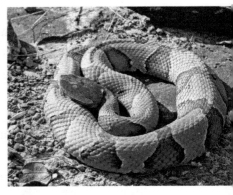

COPPERHEAD
Creeping Things/Shutterstock

TICKS These arachnids are often found in brush and tall grass, where they wait to hitch a ride on warm-blooded passersby. Adult ticks are most active April–May and again in October–November. The black-legged tick, or deer tick (left), is the primary carrier of Lyme disease.

When hiking, wear light-colored clothing to make it easier to spot ticks before they can burrow in. Afterward, visually check hair, the back of the neck, armpits, and socks. Run your clothes through a dryer cycle to kill any stragglers, and take a moment during your posthike shower to do a more complete check of your entire body. Use tweezers to remove attached ticks: grasp the tick close to the skin, and pull it straight out rather than twisting. Thoroughly clean the bite and your hands with disinfectant solution or soap and water. If you later feel ill or a red, ringlike rash develops around the bite, see a doctor.

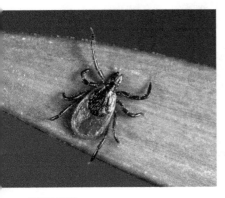

DEER TICK
Jim Gathany/Centers for Disease Control and Prevention (public domain)

Hunting

Separate rules, regulations, and licenses govern the various hunting types and related seasons. You may wish to avoid hiking during the big-game seasons, usually in November and December, when the woods suddenly seem filled with orange and camouflage. In East Tennessee, you may encounter hunters in **Cherokee National Forest** and other wildlife-management areas through which hiking trails travel.

Trail Etiquette

Always treat the trail, wildlife, and your fellow hikers with respect. Here are some reminders.

★ *Plan ahead in order to be self-sufficient at all times.* For example, carry necessary supplies for changes in weather or other conditions.

★ *Hike on open trails only.*

★ *Respect trail and road closures.* Avoid possible trespassing on private land (ask if not sure), and obtain all permits and authorization as required. Also, leave gates as you found them or as marked.

★ *Be courteous to other hikers, bikers, equestrians,* and others you may encounter on the trails.

★ *Never spook wild animals or pets.* An unannounced approach, a sudden movement, or a loud noise startles most critters, and a surprised animal can be dangerous to you, to others, and to itself. Give animals plenty of space.

★ *Observe any* YIELD *signs you encounter.* Typically, they advise hikers to yield to horses, and bikers to yield to both horses and hikers. Observing common courtesy on hills, hikers and bikers yield to any uphill traffic. When encountering mounted riders or horsepackers, hikers can courteously step off the trail, on the downhill side if possible. Calmly greet riders before they reach you, and don't dart behind trees. (You'll seem less spooky to the horse if it can see and hear you.) Also, don't pet a horse unless you're invited to do so.

★ *Leave only footprints.* Be sensitive to the ground beneath you. This also means staying on the existing trail and not blazing any new trails.

★ *Be sure to pack out what you pack in.* No one likes to see the trash someone else has left behind.

Tips on Enjoying Hiking in Greater Knoxville

Before you go, read the hike descriptions in this book. Note the website and phone number at the beginning of each hike profile, visit the website of the intended hiking destination, and call ahead if you have unanswered questions.

Investigate different areas of East Tennessee. The Smokies is the hiking kingpin, no doubt, but expand your horizons literally with a trip to the

Cumberland Plateau, or check out a local greenway or some of the fine local state parks. Try new places. Take a chance and make a new adventure instead of trying to re-create the same one over and over. You'll be pleasantly surprised to see so many distinct landscapes in greater Knoxville.

Take your time along the trails. Pace yourself. Our area is filled with wonders both big and small. Don't rush past a tiny salamander to get to that overlook. Stop and smell the wildflowers. Go ahead and take a seat on a trailside rock. Peer into a stream to find secretive fish. Take pictures. Make memories. Don't miss the trees for the forest.

We can't always schedule our free time when we want, but try to hike during the week and avoid the traditional holidays if possible. Trails that are packed in the summer are often clear during the colder months. If you are hiking on a busy day, go early in the morning to enhance your chances of seeing wildlife. The trails really clear out during rainy times, which you might consider for your outing; however, don't hike during a thunderstorm.

BIG RIDGE STATE PARK PRESENTS AQUATIC SPLENDOR. *(See Hike 14, page 80.)*

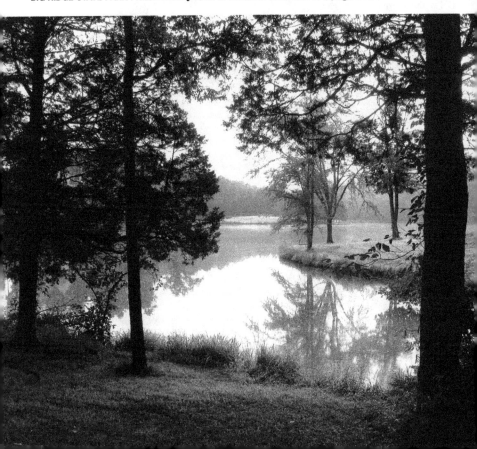

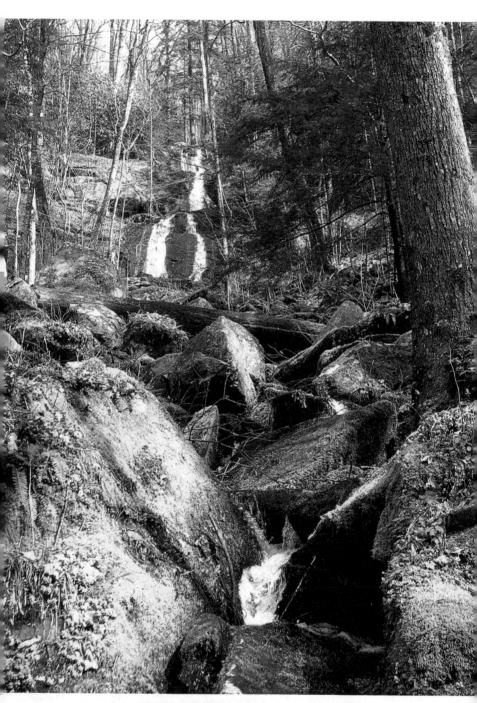

FERN BRANCH FALLS *(See Hike 37, page 184.)*

Map Legend

Featured trail   Alternate trail   Directional arrows   Off-map pointer

Interstate   Major road   Minor road

Unpaved road   Boardwalk   Stairs

Power line   Railroad   Borderline

Park/forest   Water body   River/creek/intermittent stream

𝑘 Baseball field	🏌 Golf course	🚻 Restrooms
🚤 Boat launch	H Hospital	Scenic viewpoint
✕ Bridge	✕ Mine/quarry	⊏ Shelter
△ Campground	𝟙 Monument	○ Spring
𝟙 Cemetery	▲ Overlook	Store
𝑘 Church	P Parking	Swimming
Dam	Pavilion	𝑅 Tower
Fishing	▲ Peak	Tunnel
Gate	Picnic table	// Waterfall
● General point of interest	Ranger station	

Knoxville (Hikes 1–6)

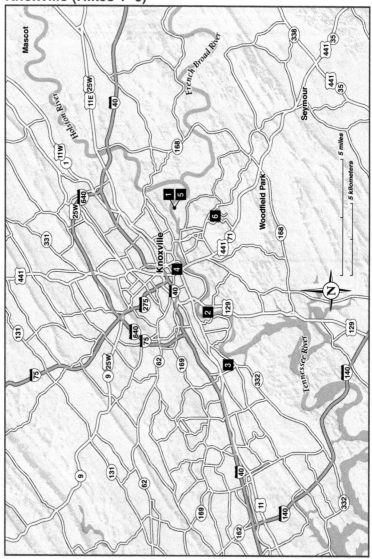

Knoxville

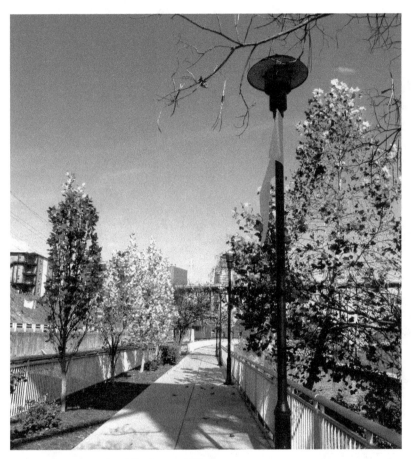

NEYLAND GREENWAY *(See Hike 4, page 34.)*

Ijams Nature Center Loop

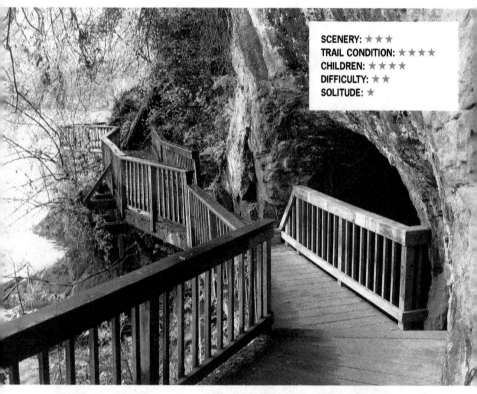

SCENERY: ★ ★ ★
TRAIL CONDITION: ★ ★ ★ ★
CHILDREN: ★ ★ ★ ★
DIFFICULTY: ★ ★
SOLITUDE: ★

ENJOY THE BOARDWALK, WHICH SQUEEZES BETWEEN A BLUFF AND THE TENNESSEE RIVER.

GPS TRAILHEAD COORDINATES: N35° 57.335' W83° 52.096'

DISTANCE & CONFIGURATION: 3-mile double loop with spurs

HIKING TIME: 1.8 hours

HIGHLIGHTS: Environmental education, river views, history

ELEVATION: 835' at low point, 1,160' at high point

ACCESS: No fees, permits, or passes required; grounds open daily, 8 a.m.–sunset

MAPS: Ijams Trail Map, USGS *Shooks Gap*

FACILITIES: Restrooms, water fountain at Ijams Visitor Center

WHEELCHAIR ACCESS: Yes, on nearby Universal Trail

COMMENTS: Ijams is dog friendly.

CONTACTS: Ijams Nature Center, 865-577-4717, ijams.org

Overview

This hike at Ijams uses a series of hiker-only trails to make a pair of loops. Leave the worth-a-visit visitor center to bisect wooded hills and then reach Mead's Quarry. Here, you circle around the lake left over after marble-mining operations ceased. The circuit makes a big climb above the quarry, reaching a pair of overlooks. It then heads toward the Tennessee River, making a side trip to Toll Creek, then explores a bluff-side boardwalk over the river. See Maude Moore's Cave; pass by a wildflower-rich hillside near Otter Island, and then climb back to the nature center.

Route Details

Now in its seventh decade, Ijams Nature Center continues to be a popular destination for Knoxville residents. Originally the home and property of Alice Ijams in the early 1900s, the grounds were opened to the public in 1965 by the City of Knoxville. Through the years the park has expanded in size, environmental-education opportunities, and trail mileage. Today, the nature center uses nearly 260 acres to display and protect this urban green space. On this hike you will cover most of the hiker-only trails. On return visits, you can make other loops of your own, altering routes to accommodate your companions. The spring wildflowers are one reason to visit, but you will find something worth seeing any time of year.

Facing the visitor center with your back to a nearby pavilion, head right, east, to pass under a covered trailhead. Walk left a few feet, then turn right on South Cove Trail. Shortly, pass the Tower Trail on your left, then the Beech Trail on your right, while hiking beneath a second-growth hardwood forest. Descend to reach the wide River Trail at 0.3 mile. Turn right here, toward Mead's Quarry, and intersect the Will Skelton Greenway (see Hike 5, page 38).

Turn left to travel south on the asphalt greenway for a short distance, then turn right to carefully cross Island Home Avenue, entering the Mead's Quarry site. This area was mined for pink marble, used in buildings throughout the United States, from the 1890s to the 1970s. Water naturally filled the quarry after it was dug out, leaving an attractive lake backed by tall granite bluffs.

This hike picks up Tharpe Trace, curving around the east side of the lake. Briefly follow an old road, then veer right onto a dirt path, climbing to reach Stanton Cemetery. Note the marked and unmarked graves, with some

Ijams Nature Center Loop

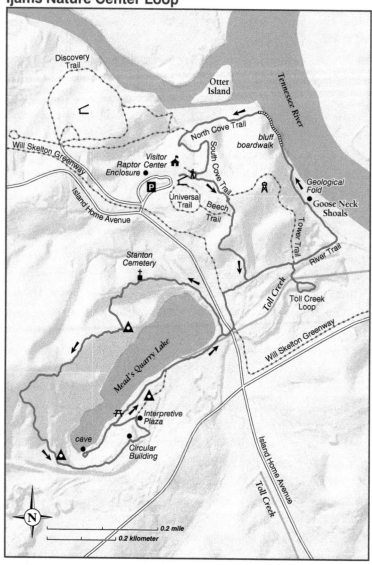

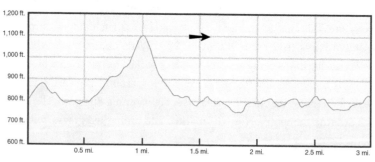

of the tombstones hand-inscribed. Many of those interred actually worked at Mead's Quarry.

Less energetic hikers may skip this loop, but for a beautiful vista, continue climbing beyond the cemetery to an overlook at 0.8 mile. Look down on the blue water and scan the surrounding hills and homes beyond the nature center. Reach a high point of 1,160 feet at 1 mile. You just climbed 330 feet from Island Home Avenue. Its downhill from here.

The downgrade eases at 1.2 miles, where another overlook allows a long view of the lake. Look for old brick, cut block, and cables—relics from when this quarry was in operation. Pass a spur trail to a circular structure that is painted to resemble a bird. Proceed to a flat area known as the Interpretive Plaza and reach a trail junction at 1.4 miles. An alluring lake overlook and picnic shelter stand to the right, but this hike goes left, southwest, on Pink Marble Trace.

Shortly, you'll reach 25-acre Mead's Quarry Lake. (By the way, boats can be rented in season for paddling the lake. No private boats allowed.) There is also a designated swimming area. Stay left, heading for Mead's Quarry Cave, which features a stream flowing into Mead's Quarry Lake. Stairs and a boardwalk allow you to peer inside the home of endangered cave species such as bats and salamanders. Pink Marble Trace travels along the water, passing aquatic access paths. This part of the hike demonstrates how to turn an eyesore into an eyepleaser. What once was an abandoned quarry is now the centerpiece of a trail network. Leave the quarry site and return to Island Home Avenue at 1.9 miles.

The Will Skelton Greenway, just across the road, takes you back to the River Trail, where you turn right. Walk northeast on the River Trail and make a four-way junction at 2.1 miles. Take the Toll Creek Loop right as it drops to a boardwalk, crossing Toll Creek twice. The urban stream has its beauty—and garbage, strewn by litterbugs and then washed into the creek. Back at the four-way junction, turn right and take the River Trail to the Tennessee River, passing a stairway leading up to an interesting geological formation—folded rock strata with the layers easily visible. At 2.5 miles, join my favorite highlight: a bluff boardwalk overhanging the Tennessee River. Take it to work your way around the steep bluff. River views are extensive. Peer into Maude Moore's Cave, its two entrances now barred.

Curve away from the Tennessee, then come near Otter Island to reach a trail junction at 2.8 miles. Stay left with the North Cove Trail, ascending a wildflower-covered hill. Come behind the nature center. and complete your loop at 3 miles.

Nearby Attractions

The park also features 9 miles of mountain biking trails located south and west of Mead's Quarry Lake, with accesses on Island Home Boulevard and Aberdeen Lane. These trails are open to hikers.

Directions

From the intersection of Cumberland Avenue and Gay Street in downtown Knoxville, drive south over the Tennessee River on the Gay Street Bridge to reach a traffic light. Keep straight at the light, now on Sevier Avenue. Travel Sevier Avenue for 0.6 mile, then stay left on Island Home Avenue as Sevier Avenue curves right over railroad tracks. Stay on Island Home Avenue for 2 miles to reach Ijams Nature Center on your left.

A VIEW INTO MEAD'S QUARRY LAKE

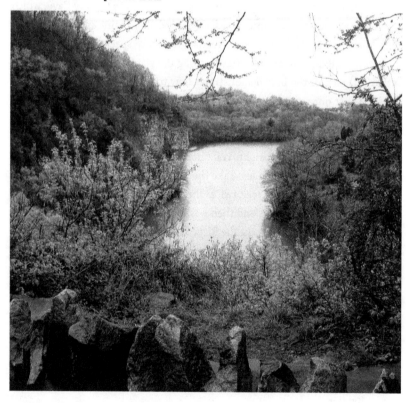

Knox/Blount Greenway

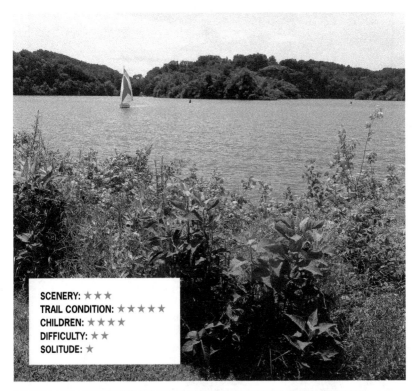

SCENERY: ★ ★ ★
TRAIL CONDITION: ★ ★ ★ ★ ★
CHILDREN: ★ ★ ★ ★
DIFFICULTY: ★ ★
SOLITUDE: ★

BOATERS CAN LAUNCH THEIR BOATS AT MARINE PARK, BY THIS HIKE'S TRAILHEAD.

GPS TRAILHEAD COORDINATES: N35° 55.764' W83° 57.047'

DISTANCE & CONFIGURATION: 3.6-mile out-and-back

HIKING TIME: 1.7 hours

OUTSTANDING FEATURES: Tennessee River views

ELEVATION: 820' at trailhead, 840' at high point

ACCESS: No fees, permits, or passes required; open daily, sunrise–sunset

MAPS: Knox/Blount Greenway Corridor map (see website below), USGS *Knoxville*

FACILITIES: Picnic tables, boat ramp at trailhead

WHEELCHAIR ACCESS: Yes, entire trail

COMMENTS: Bring binoculars for boat-watching.

CONTACTS: City of Knoxville, Tennessee Parks & Recreation, 865-215-4311, tinyurl.com/knoxblountgreenway

Knox/Blount Greenway

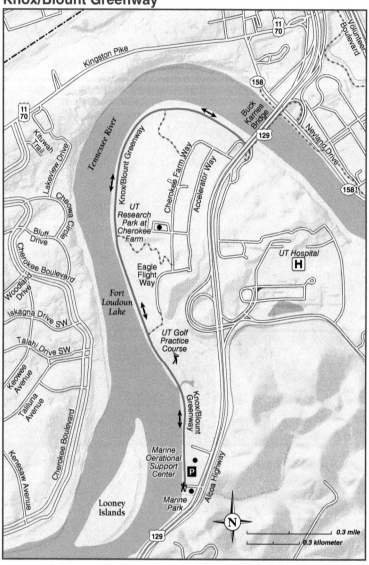

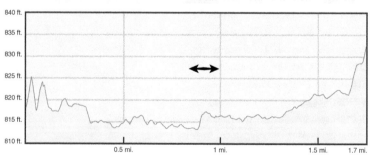

Overview

This greenway runs astride the Tennessee River with views of the river and the Sequoyah Hills and bluffs beyond. The level trail leads upstream from Marine Park to the J. E. "Buck" Karnes Bridge and offers a fast and surprisingly scenic venue where you can also enjoy watching boats on the river as well as fine homes lining the far bluff and shores.

Route Details

This hike travels through less developed lands mostly owned by the University of Tennessee (UT), presenting an opportunity to walk through a parklike shoreline atmosphere along the Tennessee River. The hike overlooks the Looney Islands at its beginning and follows the curve of the river, ending with you admiring buildings of the university.

Established in 2015, the segment of the Knox/Blount Greenway covered by this hike is living up to its name, linking Knox and Blount Counties as construction work on Alcoa Highway continues. The ultimate dream is a trail all the way to Townsend and Great Smoky Mountains National Park. On the other end, near this hike's end, the Knox/Blount Greenway connects to the greater Knoxville greenway system, crossing the Tennessee River on a dedicated pedestrian/bike path over the Buck Karnes Bridge, linking to the Neyland Greenway, which in turn links to a host of other greenways coursing through Knoxville.

Specifically, the Knox/Blount Greenway travels through UT's Cherokee Farm property, which is currently being developed as an "innovation campus" called the UT Research Park. Spur trails lead from the riverside greenway to various parking areas up on the hill where the innovation campus stands. Start the adventure by leaving north from Marine Park, passing between the river and the U.S. Marine operational support center next door. Scan the river for the Looney Islands. Beyond, the stately manors of the Sequoyah Hills neighborhood line the river. After 0.3 mile, come along the UT golf practice area used by the men's and women's golf teams. Just ahead, bridge a little creek flowing into the big Tennessee River. In many places a screen of trees lines the river. In others you gain a clear look at the waterway and beyond.

Before the Tennessee Valley Authority (TVA) was established in the 1930s, the river along which you now walk was called the Holston River. Back then, the Holston ended at its confluence with the Little Tennessee River about

50 miles downstream of Knoxville, and that was where the Tennessee River officially began. But when the TVA was authorized by Congress, its headquarters were mandated to be on the Tennessee River. The TVA wanted its headquarters in Knoxville, which at the time was on the Holston, so it decided to move the official beginning of the Tennessee River upstream to the confluence of the French Broad and Holston—which just happened to be upstream of Knoxville. Thus the TVA got its headquarters on the Tennessee River and the Holston lost 50 miles of waterway. *Hmmm* . . .

At 0.6 mile, the first of three spur trails leads up to part of the UT innovation campus. These side paths can provide additional mileage or new trail if you become a regular hiker here, as many local residents have—the past 20 years have seen phenomenal growth in greenways for Knoxville.

Exactly what is a greenway? A greenway is a linear park—a corridor of protected land overlaid with a path. Greenways can be asphalt, gravel, or mulch and often follow creeks or lakes, as this greenway does. Greenways also utilize former railroad rights-of-way, utility rights-of-way, or already established parklands linking two parks together. Sometimes, new land is purchased for greenways or an easement is granted, as was the case with this trail. Greenways are most often linear but can be a loop confined to one park; although primarily used for recreational travel, they can also be used by commuters.

These parks appeal across the human spectrum. You will see runners, in-line skaters, mothers pushing their newborns in strollers, and couples strolling hand in hand. Not surprisingly, bicyclists love greenways.

Greenways also provide urban wildlife habitats and travel corridors, allowing overall larger territories for wildlife to exist. They enhance urban aesthetics, improving quality of place, as well as the property values of adjacent lands. When it comes to public safety, they are likely to attract alert citizens versus criminals seeking to do harm; plus, they can reduce stormwater runoff and flooding. Greater Knoxville is growing fast. Hopefully, area greenways will continue to grow along with it.

The Knox/Blount Greenway continues north. Mown paths parallel the trail, in case you want to make a grassy hike. At 0.9 mile, a winding path leads up to another trail access at the UT Research Park. The greenway soon curves east as a bluff rises on the far side of the river, where historic Bleak House and Crescent Bend stand among the row of impressive manses. At 1.4 miles, another spur climbs to the innovation campus. Now you have turned northeast and are facing the main UT campus and adjacent Fort Sanders area.

Continue until you reach the shade of the Alcoa Highway Bridge (Buck Karnes Bridge) at 1.8 miles; then you can turn around—not a step before. If you want to continue across the river, proceed under the bridge; then a right-leading spur takes you to a protected path astride the bridge. The span offers wonderful but noisy views of the waterway and the UT campus beyond, as well as Cherokee Bluff.

Nearby Attractions

Marine Park has a boat launch for paddlers and boaters, in addition to a picnic area and popular bank-fishing spot.

Directions

From Exit 386B off I-40 just west of downtown Knoxville, take US 129 South (Alcoa Highway) for 2.7 miles to the right-turn entrance to Marine Park (2201 Alcoa Highway), just after the Marine Operational Support Center. This section of the Knox Blount Greenway starts from the north end of the park's parking area.

THE GREENWAY RUNS ALONG THE TENNESSEE RIVER.

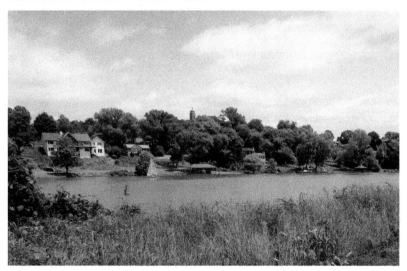

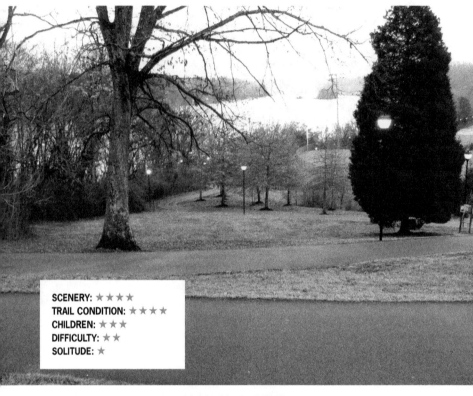

SCENERY: ★ ★ ★ ★
TRAIL CONDITION: ★ ★ ★ ★
CHILDREN: ★ ★ ★
DIFFICULTY: ★ ★
SOLITUDE: ★

VIEWS OF THE TENNESSEE RIVER STRETCH TO THE HORIZON.

GPS TRAILHEAD COORDINATES: N35° 55.430' W83° 59.397'

DISTANCE & CONFIGURATION: 2.1-mile loop

HIKING TIME: 1.2 hours

HIGHLIGHTS: Incredible river and mountain views, loop greenway

ELEVATION: 920' at trailhead, 815' along river

ACCESS: No fees, passes, or permits required; open daily, sunrise–sunset

MAPS: Lakeshore Greenway map (see website below), USGS *Knoxville*

FACILITIES: Restrooms and drinking fountains near ball fields

WHEELCHAIR ACCESS: Yes, for entire trail

COMMENTS: Loop has no other greenway connections.

CONTACTS: Knoxville Parks and Recreation, Lakeshore Park; 865-215-4311; knoxvilletn.gov

Overview

The river and mountain views will impress first-time visitors to this 60-acre park, located astride a state-run mental-health institute. Start atop a hill overlooking the Tennessee River, then drop alongside Knoxville's master waterway, gaining aquatic vistas before turning up Fourth Creek and exploring the attractive, rolling grounds of the historic facility.

Route Details

The notion of creating a park on the grounds of a downsized mental-health facility was hard to swallow for some, but it has turned out to be a great idea. Lakeshore is a state-run center that serves the mental health needs of East Tennesseans. It opened as East Tennessee Hospital for the Insane in 1886, then became known as Eastern State Mental Hospital. The place had a less-than-sterling reputation, as mentally ill Tennesseans were housed on the prisonlike grounds with little rehabilitation taking place. Such were the times, and the bad rap stayed long after the place was downsized and modernized. The grounds themselves, located on a hill above and along Fourth Creek, are stunning and today would go for big bucks. Lakeshore Park was established in 1995, and this 2.1-mile greenway runs along the perimeter of the grounds. The asphalt trail is used by walkers and joggers who want to enjoy not only the views but also the hills that add extra zing to their exercise regimen. The trail also travels past many buildings of the institute, some of which are not being used.

Leave the parking area, heading east along a hill. First-rate panoramas of East Tennessee open in moments, including a long sweep of the Tennessee River, revealing the Smoky Mountains rising over the water. What a view! Park benches beckon here, and a few cedars border the track. At 0.1 mile, the Lakeshore Greenway switchbacks off the hill under planted oaks and cedars to saddle alongside the Tennessee River, which is dammed as Fort Loudoun Lake at this point. The path is mostly open to the sky overhead as you pass beside ball fields. At 0.7 mile, the path turns west, away from the river and along the Fourth Creek embayment. Look for waterfowl in the shallows. The trail is marked in quarter-mile increments as it continues to skirt the property's outer edge. Pass planted sycamores lining the track. The entire greenway is lighted, allowing for sunrise and sunset walks, if you are so inclined.

Lakeshore Greenway

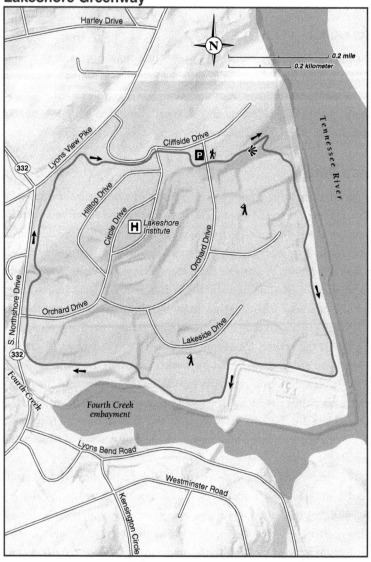

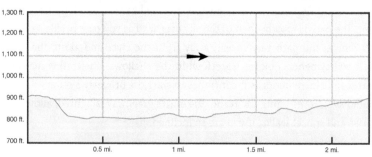

At 1.1 miles, the trail makes a short but very steep incline, only to level out again. Cruise past institute buildings, and meet up with Northshore Drive at 1.3 miles. The Lakeshore Greenway continues its loop, now heading north. Bisect an alternate property entrance at 1.5 miles. Get ready for a good hill, which then levels off. Ahead, the white stone memorials of East Tennessee State Veterans Cemetery are visible across Lyons View Pike. The cemetery for Lakeshore is nearby, where patients were interred after they passed away. (At one time Lakeshore was also used for patients with illnesses such as tuberculosis, as well as what is today known as Alzheimer's. Most of the 4,000 Lakeshore internee graves are unmarked.)

Continue an uptick while turning away from Lyons View. At 1.9 miles, come alongside the park entrance road. The greenway seemingly stops, but cross a parking lot and then rejoin the path as it curves under a magnolia tree to complete the loop at 2.1 miles.

Directions

From Exit 383 off I-40 in Knoxville, follow Papermill Drive 0.3 mile to reach Northshore Drive. Turn left, southbound, on Northshore to cross Kingston Pike. Keep south beyond Kingston Pike 0.8 mile to reach Lyons View Pike at a light. Turn left on Lyons View, and follow it 0.3 mile to the right turn into Lakeshore Institute, where a sign indicates LAKESHORE GREENWAY. Enter the grounds, passing a stop sign at 0.2 mile. Continue beyond the sign, passing buildings on your right to reach the greenway parking area, also on your right.

Neyland Greenway

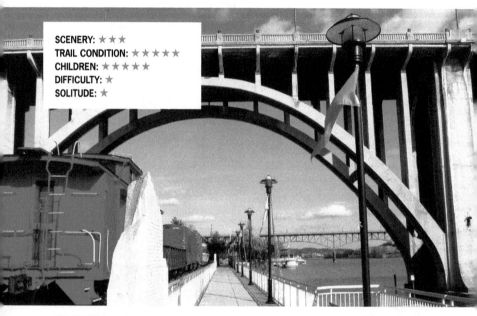

VOLUNTEER LANDING IS A POINT OF PRIDE FOR KNOXVILLIANS.

SCENERY: ★ ★ ★
TRAIL CONDITION: ★ ★ ★ ★ ★
CHILDREN: ★ ★ ★ ★
DIFFICULTY: ★
SOLITUDE: ★

GPS TRAILHEAD COORDINATES: N35° 35.651' W84° 12.510'

DISTANCE & CONFIGURATION: 3-mile out-and-back

HIKING TIME: 1.5 hours

HIGHLIGHTS: City views, lake views

ELEVATION: 835' at trailhead, 850' at high point

ACCESS: No fees, permits, or passes required; open daily, sunrise–sunset

MAPS: Neyland Greenway map (see website below), USGS *Knoxville*

FACILITIES: Water, restrooms, riverside benches at trailhead

WHEELCHAIR ACCESS: Yes, for entire greenway

CONTACTS: Knoxville Parks and Recreation, 865-215-4311, knoxvilletn.gov/neylandgreenway

Overview

This downtown greenway starts at Volunteer Landing, off Neyland Drive astride the Tennessee River, where an alluring trailhead makes for a great place to relax before or after your hike. Head west on the greenway along the river before tunneling under Neyland Drive at the Second Creek Greenway. Continue down Neyland Drive, passing iconic Neyland Stadium before returning to the river to soak in views of the Cherokee Bluffs across the water and then backtracking. Keep in mind this is an urban trek involving a road crossing and city sounds and sights. Also, this greenway connects to other trails, allowing you to add mileage to this outing.

Route Details

Neyland Greenway is a scenic urban path and an important connector that links several other paved paths in Knoxville's ever-expanding city trail system, including the James White Greenway, Morningside Greenway, Second Creek Greenway, Third Creek Greenway, and Knox/Blount Greenway. This trek starts at downtown's Volunteer Landing, one of many developed areas along Neyland Greenway; the brick structure overlooking the Tennessee River has restrooms, water, and benches, all designed for enjoying the riverside scenery. Restaurants and entertainment are all within easy walking distance. Downtown Knoxville is up the hill from the river.

Pick up the greenway and travel west, away from Calhoun's Restaurant. Enjoy views of the Tennessee River and the land rising across the water. Soon enter an area with many artsy fountains where kids play in summer. The concrete walkway is lined with attractive iron railings and lampposts, and interpretive signage delivers historical vignettes detailing Knoxville's longtime relationship with the Tennessee River—the reason for the city's being here in the first place. The stuff is really fascinating. Take the time to read up on and visualize the many incarnations of the area where you walk.

Railroad tracks, Neyland Drive, and boats on the river remind you this area has long been a transportation corridor. The greenway is yet another venue as walkers, bikers, and in-line skaters ply the concrete track. Volunteers fans access it to attend University of Tennessee (UT) sporting events. Boat landings are used by visitors and the Vol Navy, an impromptu flotilla of UT football devotees who voyage the river to see the Big Orange in action. Pass under the historic arched Henley Street Bridge and then under a utilitarian railroad bridge at 0.3 mile. Ahead, come to an intersection. Here, the Neyland Greenway curves left over the river at the UT Rowing Club Building, then tunnels under Neyland Drive along Second Creek. Once on the north side of Neyland Drive, you reach

Neyland Greenway

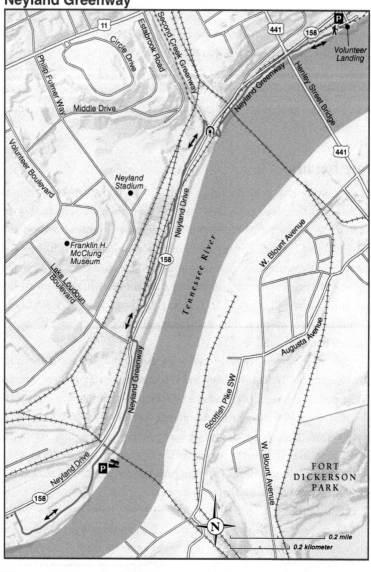

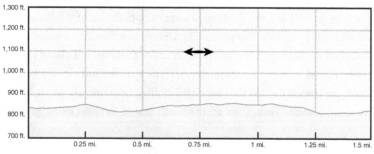

a greenway intersection. Here, the Second Creek Greenway heads north along Second Creek to World's Fair Park.

You take the now-asphalt Neyland Greenway up the north side of Neyland Drive and pass Neyland Stadium, home of UT Volunteers football. Keep along the drive, passing in the shadow of Thompson-Boling Arena (where the men's and women's teams play basketball) to reach Lake Loudoun Boulevard and a traffic light at 0.9 mile. Cross Neyland Drive at the crosswalk, then resume the greenway, now back along the Tennessee River. Enjoy views of boaters and rowers on nice days. At 1.2 miles, travel under another railroad bridge. The path then turns away from Neyland Drive, passing an alternate parking area with just a few spaces, as well as the public Neyland Drive boat ramp.

The greenway then circles behind a City of Knoxville water treatment plant. A wooden boardwalk extends over rock riprap on the water. The Cherokee Bluffs rise 250 feet across the river. This is a favorite spot for river lovers. At 1.5 miles, the Neyland Greenway returns to Neyland Drive. This is a good place to turn around, but you can continue along the greenway for 0.4 mile to reach the Third Creek Greenway, while the Knox/Blount Greenway is another half mile distant. Also, if you want to extend your trek in the other direction, the Neyland Greenway heads east from Volunteer Landing, where you started, to meet the James White Greenway, which heads north to Morningside Park.

Nearby Attractions

The **Women's Basketball Hall of Fame** is just down the road. Check out the history of women's basketball through the decades in this city where the Tennessee Lady Volunteers continue to set the standard of greatness. For more information visit wbhof.com.

Directions

From Exit 388A off I-40 in Knoxville, take James White Parkway southbound; then, in about 0.5 mile, veer right onto the Neyland Drive exit, continuing south. Neyland Drive soon follows the Tennessee River. Turn left into Volunteer Landing at a traffic light signed for Walnut Street. Cross the railroad tracks and turn right for parking (the left turn is for parking at Calhoun's restaurant).

5

Will Skelton Greenway

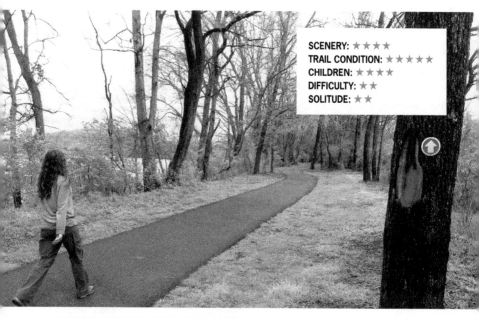

SCENERY: ★ ★ ★ ★
TRAIL CONDITION: ★ ★ ★ ★ ★
CHILDREN: ★ ★ ★ ★
DIFFICULTY: ★ ★
SOLITUDE: ★ ★

TREKKING THE GREENWAY IN EARLY SPRING

GPS TRAILHEAD COORDINATES: N35° 57.335' W83° 52.099'

DISTANCE & CONFIGURATION: 4.2-mile out-and-back

HIKING TIME: 2.2 hours

HIGHLIGHTS: River views, wildlife management area

ELEVATION: 865' at trailhead, 845' at turnaround point

ACCESS: No fees, permits, or passes required; open daily, sunrise–sunset

MAPS: Will Skelton Greenway map (see website below), USGS *Shooks Gap*

FACILITIES: Restrooms and water fountain at Ijams Nature Center

WHEELCHAIR ACCESS: Yes, for entire trail

COMMENTS: This greenway is part of the larger Urban Wilderness Loop.

CONTACTS: Knoxville Parks & Recreation, 865-215-4311, tinyurl.com/willskeltongreenway

Overview

This paved trek leaves Ijams Nature Center using the Will Skelton Greenway
to enter Forks of the River Wildlife Management Area, a natural setting of
woodland and meadow interspersed with additional trails open to hikers but

dominated by mountain bikers. Cruise along the inception of the Tennessee River, and then curve up the French Broad River to end at a bluff offering elevated views of the French Broad and beyond. Some hills add to the challenge, while creeks add more watery scenery.

Route Details

Will Skelton is a well-known conservationist icon of Knoxville's parks, greenways, and general outdoors scene. Active both locally and nationally in the Sierra Club, he was an instrumental part of the Cherokee National Forest Wilderness Coalition, which helped set aside roadless areas in Tennessee's only national forest. He even edited a book about the trails of the Cherokee. A retired lawyer, Skelton championed building greenways in Knoxville, serving as the chairman of the Knoxville Greenways Commission, so it is only fitting that such a scenic path would be named for him.

The Will Skelton Greenway, popular with walkers, bicyclists, and joggers, begins at Island Home Park, then travels east to reach Ijams Nature Center, where this hike picks up the path (also see Hike 1, page 20). Enjoy traveling through nature center property, and then bisect a brief section of civilization to enter the wildlife management area, which presents a natural scene for you to enjoy.

From the nature center entrance, head southeast on a 10-foot-wide asphalt track. Island Home Avenue is to your right. The trail immediately passes a solar-energy capture station that helps power the Ijams Nature Center visitor building. Immediately enter lush woods, then make a downward curve. Traverse an old railroad track near Mead's Quarry, which is visible to your right (southwest); then, at 0.4 mile, bridge Toll Creek, which gurgles its way to meet the Tennessee River. At this point, you will leave Ijams Nature Center property.

The trail then turns sharply east as it parallels McClure Lane. Here, the path exhibits characteristics more typical of an urban greenway, a track paralleling houses and businesses. However, this section is short-lived as, at 0.8 mile, the greenway leaves McClure Lane and bridges a creek to come alongside the Tennessee River.

Enter the Forks of the River Wildlife Management Area (WMA), managed by the Tennessee Wildlife Resources Agency but increasingly used by nonhunting outdoor enthusiasts. The name Forks of the River refers to the three rivers that come together at this point. The French Broad River has cut east through the mountains from North Carolina, while the Holston River has come from the

Will Skelton Greenway

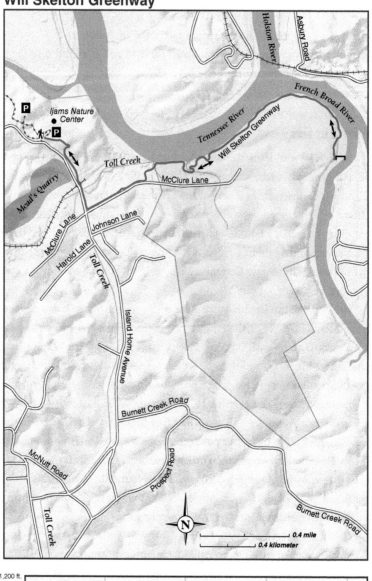

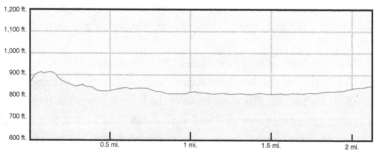

coal country of southwestern Virginia. Both rivers travel a fair distance through the Volunteer State, and it is here that their waters meet to form the Tennessee River. The WMA presents a green landscape of open fields and cedar and hardwood forests, along with wetlands and the riparian zone that borders the Tennessee and French Broad Rivers. It is amazing that this 605-acre tract of wilderness lies so close to downtown Knoxville. You may see wildlife that calls this area home. Hikers will commonly spot deer and wild turkeys, while birders can enjoy not only songbirds but also shorebirds along the river and raptors overhead. Birders have counted more than 175 species at Forks of the River WMA. Be apprised that this wildlife management area is intermittently open to hunting between September and February, when the greenway remains open for use.

At 1 mile, bridge another stream, arguably the uppermost tributary on the entire Tennessee. Here, the trail doubles back on itself before returning to the water. Hardwoods partially shade the trail. At 1.3 miles, come alongside a large open field to your right, while a screen of vegetation lies between you and the Tennessee. Some fields are being used to grow crops for wildlife, while others have been periodically burned to restore native grasses.

At 1.6 miles, reach the vista where you can look upon the three rivers at once. See if you notice different water coloration between the French Broad and the Holston. The trail stays along the river's edge, but it has now joined the French Broad, across which barges and industry are visible. The easy, level cruise ends at 2 miles. The greenway turns away from the water and climbs to reach a bluff—the trail terminus—at 2.1 miles. Here, you can gaze up the valley of the French Broad. Pickel Island splits the river in the foreground. A resting bench beckons. From here, backtrack 2.1 miles to the trailhead to complete your hike at 4.2 miles.

Nearby Attractions

The **Knoxville Urban Wilderness Loop** makes a 12.5-mile circuit using not only the Will Skelton Greenway but also Hastie Natural Area, Marie Myers Park and Ijams Nature Center, as well as roads in places. The entire route is open to hikers and bicyclists. See visitknoxville.com/urban-wilderness for details.

Directions

From the intersection of Cumberland Avenue and Gay Street in downtown Knoxville, travel south over the Tennessee River on the Gay Street Bridge to reach the traffic light. Keep straight at the light, now on Sevier Avenue. Travel 0.6 mile on Sevier Avenue, then stay left on Island Home Avenue as Sevier curves right over railroad tracks. Stay on Island Home Avenue for 2 miles to reach Ijams Nature Center on your left. Park immediately upon entering. Pick up the Will Skelton Greenway near the Ijams entrance gate.

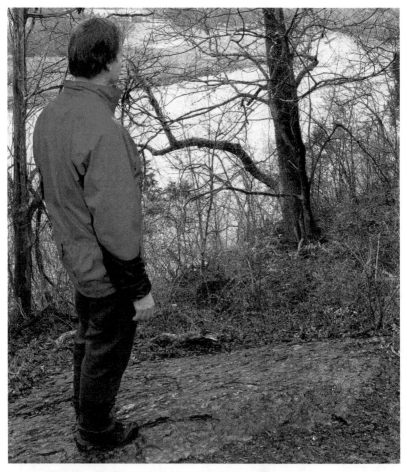

A HIKER ADMIRES THE VIEW OF THE TENNESSEE RIVER FROM A BLUFF ON THE WILL SKELTON GREENWAY.

6

William Hastie
Natural Area

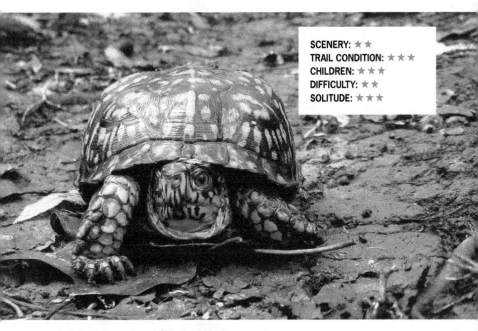

SCENERY: ★ ★
TRAIL CONDITION: ★ ★ ★
CHILDREN: ★ ★ ★
DIFFICULTY: ★ ★
SOLITUDE: ★ ★ ★

EVEN THE TURTLES LIKE KNOXVILLE'S TRAILS.

GPS TRAILHEAD COORDINATES: N35° 56.079' W83° 52.470'

DISTANCE & CONFIGURATION: 2.6-mile loop

HIKING TIME: 1.4 hours

HIGHLIGHTS: Deep woods, rock ledges and outcrops

ELEVATION: 960' at trailhead, 1,060' at high point

ACCESS: No fees, permits, or passes required; open daily, sunrise–sunset

MAPS: William Hastie Natural Area map (see website below), USGS *Shooks Gap* and *Knoxville*

FACILITIES: Picnic table and shelter

WHEELCHAIR ACCESS: None

CONTACTS: Knoxville Parks and Recreation, 865-215-4311, tinyurl.com/hastienaturalarea

Overview

This loop hike travels through a 75-acre tract of hilly wilderness located in suburban South Knoxville. Once a farm, the rugged terrain, full of rock outcrops and

William Hastie Natural Area

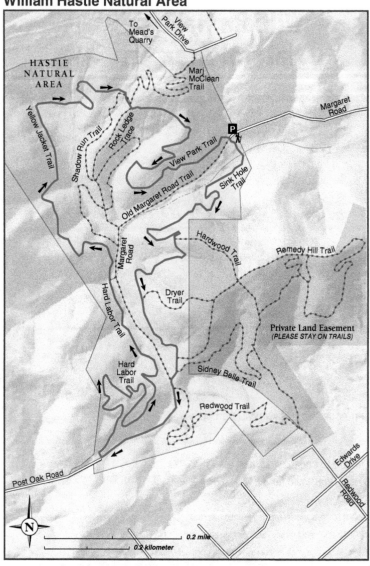

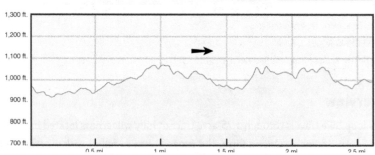

sinkholes amid dense woodland, offers nearly 7.5 miles of trails developed by a local mountain biking club. Hikers are more than welcome on the trails, which can be a quick escape for those desiring a deep-woods connection with nature.

Route Details

What a great addition to the Knoxville park system! William Hastie Natural Area contrasts greatly with typical urban parks, with their playgrounds, ball fields, and paved trails. This destination is an old hardscrabble farm reverted to wooded wildland, where natural-surface trails explore darn near every nook and cranny of the tract. You will be surprised at the steep and rugged topography— and wonder how anybody could've ever farmed it. But farm they did.

John Chandler grew up near the trailhead. In 1947, his family bought 97 acres, along with the house, which had no running water, electricity, or indoor plumbing. They collected roof runoff and drained it into a cistern for storage. The family lived off some livestock and a garden, eventually adding lights and water. Chandler was one of 13 children raised here during the 17 years they called what is now William Hastie Natural Area home. As you hike, imagine 13 kids, plus cows, pigs, and chickens, running around these now-thick woods.

Three trails split from the Margaret Road trailhead. While facing the big boulders blocking Old Margaret Road Trail, head left past the picnic shelter on Sinkhole Trail. Old Margaret Road Trail continues past the boulders, while View Park Trail (your return route) leaves to the right. The slender singletrack Sinkhole Trail shortly enters woods, where many walnut trees stand overhead. Cruise the edge of a hollow with a rocky, cedar-covered hill rising to your left.

When hiking, keep an eye and ear open for mountain bikers. They built the trails and bridges we hike. Pass over a trio of bridges at 0.2 mile. The path is generally easy to follow except where it crosses old farm roads and mountain biking trails spurring from the main route, such as the Hardwood Trail at 0.4 mile.

Meet Old Margaret Road Trail at 0.7 mile. Turn left on the gravel track, traveling the base of a hollow whereupon tulip tree–covered hills rise to a point where you wouldn't begin to guess that the park is surrounded by houses. The many sinkholes here prevent continual running water in the streambeds. At 0.8 mile, join the Hard Labor Trail as it leads acutely right. Ahead, Old Margaret Road Trail leads a short distance to meet the Post Oak neighborhood entrance to the natural area.

Continue on the Hard Labor Trail as it winds up a hillside to reach what was likely an old rock quarry. Climb into dogwoods and pines, reaching a high point at 1.1 miles. Begin a convoluted, twisted course using tight switchbacks that prevent erosion and maximize mileage in the limited space of the natural area. Note the elongated rock outcroppings and rock piles beside the path. In winter these outcrops will stand out. In spring the hollows will show off their share of wildflowers.

Descend to meet the Yellow Jacket Trail at 1.6 miles. A short path leads right to Old Margaret Road Trail. Keep straight, joining the singletrack Yellow Jacket Trail, heading north and bridging a couple of streambeds to make another trail junction at 2.2 miles. Here, the Rock Ledge Trace leaves to the right. Our loop stays left, crossing an old roadbed to pick up the singletrack View Park Trail. This path makes long, loping switchbacks down a south-facing rock, hickory, and cedar hill. Descend gently, drifting into the trailhead at 2.6 miles, to complete the loop hike.

Nearby Attractions

The natural area offers more trails in addition to the loop described. Old Margaret Road Trail cuts through the heart of the natural area and connects to all the other paths. It follows the low point of the main valley. Rock Ledge Trace winds along a hillside limestone outcrop. These trails add more loop possibilities should you want to go a different route on a second or third trip here.

Directions

From Exit 388A off I-40 east of downtown Knoxville, take James White Parkway south 3.2 miles to the Moody Avenue exit. Exit James White Parkway and then turn left, crossing over the parkway, to join Sevierville Pike. Follow Sevierville Pike 1.8 miles on a very winding road to a right turn onto Margaret Road. Follow Margaret Road 0.3 mile until it dead-ends in a parking area.

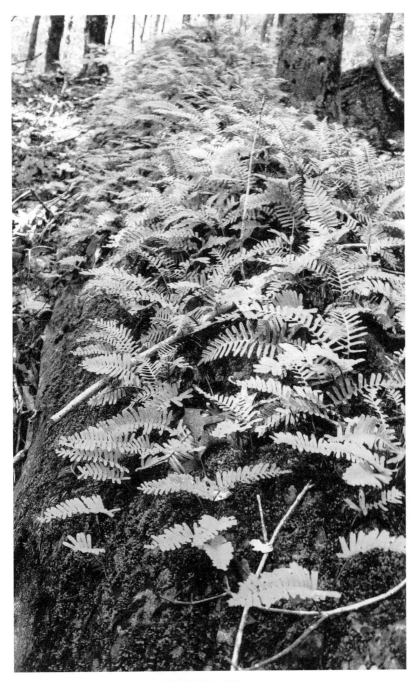

BEAUTY ABOUNDS AT WILLIAM HASTIE NATURAL AREA.

West (Hikes 7–13)

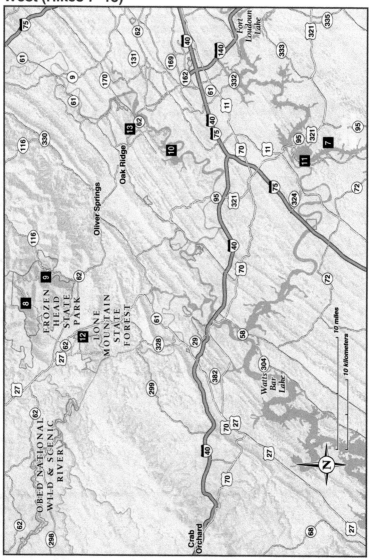

West

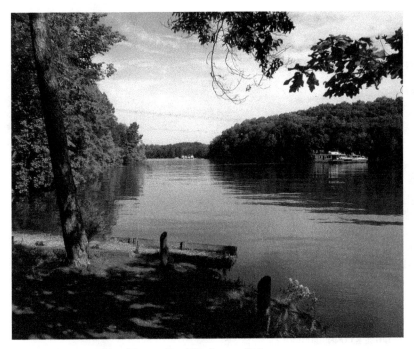

LOOKING INTO GLENDALE BRANCH *(See Hike 7, page 50.)*

7

East Lakeshore Trail

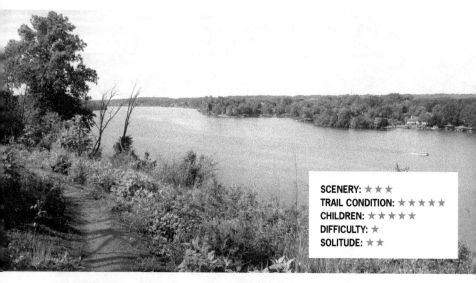

SCENERY: ★ ★ ★
TRAIL CONDITION: ★ ★ ★ ★ ★
CHILDREN: ★ ★ ★ ★ ★
DIFFICULTY: ★
SOLITUDE: ★ ★

VIEW OF TELLICO LAKE FROM A BLUFF ON THE EAST LAKESHORE TRAIL

GPS TRAILHEAD COORDINATES: N35° 43.684' W84° 13.914'

DISTANCE & CONFIGURATION: 2.5-mile balloon

HIKING TIME: 1.2 hours

OUTSTANDING FEATURES: Lakeside hiking, watery vistas, excellent trail, bluff views

ELEVATION: 820' at trailhead, 951' at high point

ACCESS: No fees, permits, or passes required; open daily, sunrise–sunset

MAPS: East Lakeshore Trail map (see Tellico Reservoir website below), USGS *Meadow*

FACILITIES: None

WHEELCHAIR ACCESS: None

COMMENTS: Trailhead accesses East Lakeshore Trail in both directions. Be careful when hiking during hunting season (late November–early January).

CONTACTS: Tennessee Valley Authority, 865-632-2101, tva.com/environment/recreation/tva-trails; Watershed Association of Tellico Reservoir, tellicowater.org/east-lakeshore-trail

Overview

Enjoy this sampler balloon loop of a 31-mile designated National Recreation Trail on the shores of Tellico Lake. Here, meander in lush forest along a protected lakeshore, then rise to a high point where distant views open. Return to lake's edge before using a shortcut to loop back to the trailhead.

Route Details

This hike will whet your appetite for more of the 31-mile East Lakeshore Trail, built on Tennessee Valley Authority (TVA) lakefront land in cooperation with the Watershed Association of Tellico Reservoir. This partnership has resulted in a beautiful and expanding trail corridor divided into nine segments, with several trailheads where hikers can access the path midroute. Most of the hikes on it are out-and-back, but our hike uses the Glendale Branch segment, which offers a shortcut trail that allows for a loop hike.

The trail system was begun in 2002 and has slowly expanded, using mostly volunteer labor. The first 30 miles were completed in 2014 after being designated a National Recreation Trail in 2012. The TVA has helped with technical support, heavy equipment, and trailhead infrastructure, as well as material for trail bridges and other construction materials. And of course, without the TVA lakefront land, the trail would never have been possible in the first place.

Today, trail maintenance is done by volunteers. (After all, Tennessee *is* the Volunteer State.) Each trailhead has a parking area and trail kiosk with a map. Using one of three trailside boat landings, boaters on Tellico Lake can pull up, get out of their watercraft, and stretch their legs on a little hike; our trail segment includes one of those boat landings. Active explorer types could even paddle to a boat landing, then hike, then paddle back to a boat ramp, executing a biathlon of sorts. Together, the waters of Tellico Lake and the segments of the East Lakeshore Trail present all sorts of possibilities.

The Glendale Branch segment shares the Glendale Trailhead with the Davis Ferry Branch segment, at mile 8 of the 31-mile linear trail. There is also an informal trailhead water access that more than one trail treader—including myself—has used to take a posthike dip. The Glendale Branch segment leaves southwest of the parking area, while the Davis Ferry Branch segment leaves northeast. Curve around a little embayment, with a pair of trail bridges spanning Glendale Branch and another tributary. After passing a private dock, the path rises a bit on steps from the water's edge.

The East Lakeshore Trail settles into a habit of mimicking the curves of the shoreline of Tellico Lake. Damming the Little Tennessee River created the 16,000-acre reservoir; at this point you are seeing only the Glendale Branch embayment of Tellico Lake. Trace the singletrack, hiker-only path through oak-dominated woods, with the water just a few feet away. At 0.3 mile, in a

East Lakeshore Trail

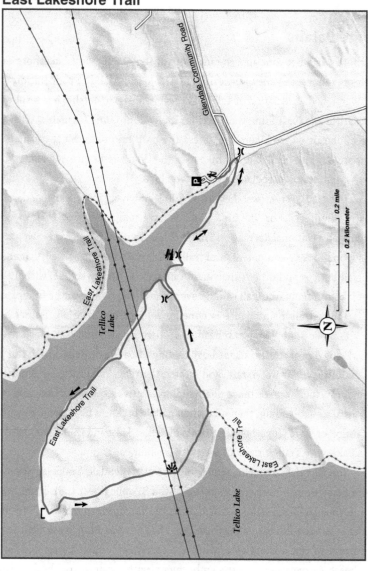

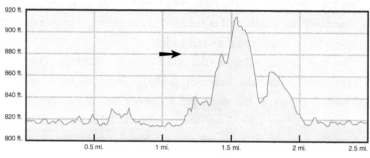

stand of pines, come to one of the East Lakeshore Trail boat landings. Even if you aren't boating, this is a good spot for taking a look at Tellico Lake.

The trail curves away from the water, bridges a creek, and then turns into a second small creek where you bridge another stream and reach an intersection at 0.5 mile. Here, the Glendale Branch Shortcut—your return route—leaves left, while the main East Lakeshore Trail keeps right, returning to the shoreline. At 0.6 mile, the trail passes under a power line before coming back along the shore. Winter views are nearly continuous, while summer hikers contend with partial vistas of the waters beyond the cedar-rich woods.

Curve out to the end of the Glendale Branch embayment, and open up to the main body of water. Reach a bench with a clear view into Tellico Lake; note the half-submerged silos rising from the water. Here, the East Lakeshore Trail turns south and you make a slight climb. At 1.5 miles, open onto a power-line cut and a fantastic view. Below you the lake and lands beyond stretch forth, with the balance of the Volunteer State opening to the west as far as the sky allows.

The trail reenters piney woods, descending back to water level to reach an intersection at 1.6 miles. Here, our return route leaves left, while the East Lakeshore Trail continues south for the Coytee Trailhead. Rise gently away from the lake, topping out where a roadbed goes both directions to wildlife clearings, and then just as gently descend, completing the loop portion of the hike at 1.9 miles. From here it's a simple 0.6-mile backtrack to the trailhead, reached at 2.5 miles. Hopefully, this trek has inspired you to tackle more of the East Lakeshore Trail.

Nearby Attractions

Tellico Lake offers boating and fishing in a gorgeous setting with the Appalachian Mountains as a backdrop.

Directions

From Exit 81 off I-75 southwest of Knoxville, take US 321 North—the road actually goes south at this point—for 7.5 miles. Turn right on TN 95 South and follow it 0.8 mile; then turn right on Glendale Community Road and follow it 1.4 miles, passing a small lakefront parking area. Continue a bit farther to the official parking area, up a little hill.

8

Frozen Head State Park:
Emory Gap Falls and DeBord Falls

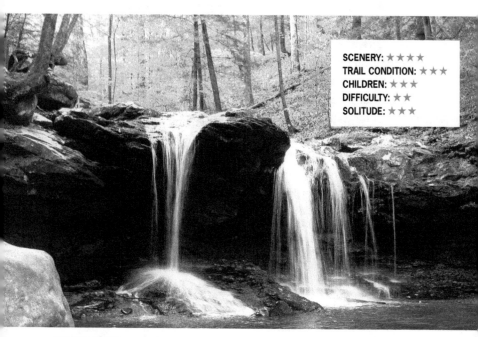

SCENERY: ★ ★ ★ ★
TRAIL CONDITION: ★ ★ ★
CHILDREN: ★ ★ ★
DIFFICULTY: ★ ★
SOLITUDE: ★ ★ ★

DEBORD FALLS

GPS TRAILHEAD COORDINATES: N36° 08.200' W84° 29.254'

DISTANCE & CONFIGURATION: 2.8-mile out-and-back

HIKING TIME: 1.8 hours

HIGHLIGHTS: Three waterfalls, Cumberland Mountains

ELEVATION: 1,520' at trailhead, 1,990' at turnaround point

ACCESS: No fees, permits, or passes required; park open daily, 7 a.m.–sunset

MAPS: Frozen Head State Park map (see website below), USGS *Fork Mountain*

FACILITIES: Restrooms, water fountains, camping, visitor center

WHEELCHAIR ACCESS: None

CONTACTS: Frozen Head State Park, 423-346-3318, tnstateparks.com/parks/frozen-head

Overview

This waterfall hike in mountainous Frozen Head State Park leads to two named cascades as it explores a rugged valley carved from the highest terrain on the entire Cumberland Plateau. The hike is easier than you might think because it follows an old roadbed most of its distance. Traveling along North Prong Flat Fork, the hike enters a wildflower-laden valley to reach DeBord Falls, complemented by a shaded pool. The ascent sharpens upon joining Emory Gap Branch, where Emory Gap Falls drops over a stone lip framed by a rock house.

Route Details

The road leading to the trailhead passes an attractive picnic area. Consider bringing a pre- or posthike meal on your Frozen Head State Park adventure. The Panther Branch parking area has a turnaround at the uppermost part, but don't park in the turnaround. Panther Branch Trail passes a trailside kiosk then immediately bridges North Prong Flat Fork. Sycamore, hemlock, and buckeye shade the stream as it flows over smooth rocks. Beech, black birch, and tulip trees rise up the valley.

Before you know it, a spur trail veers right to an unnamed waterfall spilling into Flat Fork. This modest tributary cascade tumbles off the north side of Old Mac Mountain, dropping over layers of rock before adding its flow to Flat Fork. Like many of the watercourses here at Frozen Head, this stream may run nearly dry in late summer and fall. The wide path traverses intermittent streambeds flowing off Bird Mountain to your left (north). Bird Mountain and Old Mac Mountain together create the valley through which North Prong Flat Fork flows.

Unlike most other trails at Frozen Head, this path makes for easy hiking because it follows an old jeep road, allowing you to focus on your surroundings rather than watching every footfall. Also, hikers can walk side by side, conversing as they travel. The setup is great for families. Occasional large boulders stand in the stream and among the woods around you. Small trees sometimes find a home atop the more level boulders. Keep an eye out for exposed bluffs overlooking the creek. Pass a deep, alluring pool at 0.3 mile; this is a great place for kids to play in the water and ruin their new hiking boots. The ascent picks up at 0.5 mile. Bridge a branch at 0.6 mile, then come to the spur loop leading to DeBord Falls. Here, take a short trail leading to a bluff-top overlook of the cascade. Ahead, steps lead to the base of the falls, which drops 15 feet over a jagged rock ledge into a gravel-bordered pool. A sturdy hemlock stands by in repose.

Continue up Panther Branch Trail, shortly bridging another intermittent streambed. At 0.9 mile, Panther Branch Trail leaves to the right up Panther Branch to meet North Old Mac Trail. Our hike, however, keeps straight, joining Emory Gap Trail, ascending along Emory Gap Branch. The hike still traces an old jeep road that makes a pair of switchbacks at 1.1 miles, heading deeper into the

Frozen Head State Park:
Emory Gap Falls and DeBord Falls

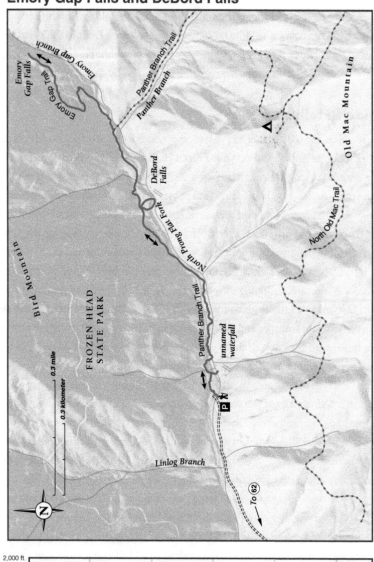

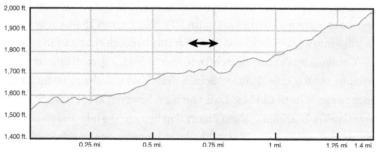

mountain valley. Bridge another intermittent streambed at 1.2 miles. Saddle alongside Emory Gap Branch as it flows through large gray boulders that obscure the flow and give the impression of a watercourse that's more rock than water.

Travel along the edge of a tall rock house. Emory Gap Falls is visible in the distance. Pick your way carefully upstream through a boulder garden bordered by the rock house on one side and Emory Gap Branch on the other. Reach the falls at 1.4 miles. Several user-created trails approach the cascade from different directions, as hikers attempt to gain the best vantage. The tall cataract spills over a rock ledge, framed on one side by the rock house and on the other by a wooded hill. Don't climb atop the falls—the mossy rocks are slick and invite disaster. Photographers will be challenged to compose the varied landscape here, with the boulder garden, rock house, surrounding woods, and waterfall. The pool below the falls is somewhat shallow, as Emory Gap Branch is a generally low-flowing creek. Your legs will enjoy the 500-foot descent back to the trailhead to complete the 2.8-mile trek much more than they liked the climb.

Nearby Attractions

Frozen Head State Park offers not only hiking but also fishing, camping, and nature study on its 21,000 acres of wildlands. Also, a segment of the Cumberland Trail travels through the park.

Directions

From Knoxville, take TN 162 (Pellissippi Parkway) toward Oak Ridge, joining TN 62 West to reach Oliver Springs. From Oliver Springs, follow TN 62 West for 13 miles and turn right onto Flat Fork Road; a sign for Morgan County Regional Correctional Facility and Frozen Head State Park alerts you to the right turn. Follow Flat Fork Road 4 miles to the entrance of Frozen Head State Park. The visitor center is on your right. Keep straight, passing the main hiker trailhead. Continue left for 1 mile beyond the main trailhead, passing the campground spur road to dead-end at the Panther Branch trailhead.

9

Frozen Head State Park:
Frozen Head Tower via Armes Gap

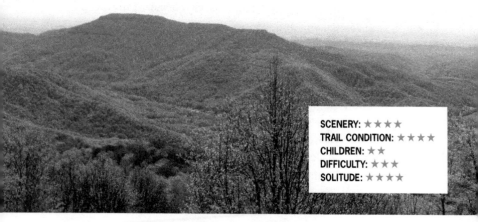

SCENERY: ★ ★ ★ ★
TRAIL CONDITION: ★ ★ ★ ★
CHILDREN: ★ ★
DIFFICULTY: ★ ★ ★
SOLITUDE: ★ ★ ★ ★

VIEWS EXTEND IN ALL DIRECTIONS FROM ATOP FROZEN HEAD.

GPS TRAILHEAD COORDINATES: N36° 06.985' W84° 26.355'

DISTANCE & CONFIGURATION: 5.4-mile out-and-back plus optional 0.8-mile out-and-back to prison mine

HIKING TIME: 4 hours

HIGHLIGHTS: 360-degree view from observation tower, historic prison mine

ELEVATION: 2,100' at trailhead, 3,324' at high point

ACCESS: No fees, permits, or passes required; park open daily, 7 a.m.–sunset

MAPS: Frozen Head State Park, USGS *Petros*

FACILITIES: None

WHEELCHAIR ACCESS: None

COMMENTS: Frozen Head State Park has more than 40 miles of hiking trails in addition to this hike.

CONTACTS: Frozen Head State Park, 423-346-3318, tnstateparks.com/parks/frozen-head

Overview

This trail takes you to one of the highest points on the Cumberland Plateau, Frozen Head Mountain, standing at 3,324 feet. Here, an observation tower allows a 360-degree view from the boundaries above Frozen Head State Park. On a clear day you can look east across the Tennessee River Valley to the Smoky Mountains and west across the Plateau as far as the clarity of the sky allows. This route is the shortest with the least amount of elevation gain, but it still climbs a solid 1,200 feet. Add a historical component by visiting the old Brushy Mountain Prison Mine on your way back.

Route Details

Lookout Tower Trail passes around a metal gate and heads southwest from Armes Gap. The gated doubletrack is open only to official vehicles. TN 116 will be on your left and is visible through the trees. You are expecting a climb, but it starts out pretty easy, picking up steam at 0.3 mile. A rich hardwood forest dominated by hickory, tulip, maple, and oak shades the gravel-and-dirt path. At 0.7 mile, reach a split. Here, Old Prison Mines Trail leads left on a level doubletrack, while Lookout Tower Trail continues to ascend. Save the Old Prison Mines Trail for your return trip after scaling Frozen Head.

On the way in, you pass the fortresslike Brushy Mountain State Prison. Established in 1896, it housed the state's most hardened criminals until it closed for good in 2009. Its most famous inmate was James Earl Ray, convicted of assassinating Martin Luther King Jr. in Memphis. Ray escaped from Brushy Mountain in the 1970s but was quickly recaptured. Today, the prison is a tourist destination open from April through December; here you can learn the story of Tennessee's most infamous prison. For more information, visit tourbrushy.com.

Beyond the intersection, Lookout Tower Trail makes a hard switchback to the right. At 0.9 mile, the path crosses over to the right (north) side of the mountain. Views open on Big Fodderstack Mountain to the east. This ridgeline marks the Tennessee Valley Divide. Streams to the north and east flow into the Cumberland River, while streams to the south and west feed the Tennessee River. Pass a small grassy clearing and keep ascending, as Frozen Head rises sharply to your left. Springs flow over rock outcrops in the forest above you.

More wintertime views open to the northeast. The trail continues curving up the mountain, turning sharply west at 1.9 miles. The climbing eases as you pass Tub Spring, enclosed in stone to your left at 2.2 miles. Drift into a major trail junction. Tub Spring Campsite lies up a small hill to your right. Lookout Tower Trail splits here. One leg heads right and downhill to the state park campground, while the other leg turns left to the crest of Frozen Head. Other trails spur from here to lace Frozen Head State Park. Stay left toward the tower, still climbing on a doubletrack. Curve around the south side of the peak. The observation tower and radio towers come into view. Reach the top of Frozen Head at 2.7 miles. Here, an old apple tree grows next to radio towers. Steps lead to an open observation

Frozen Head State Park:
Frozen Head Tower via Armes Gap

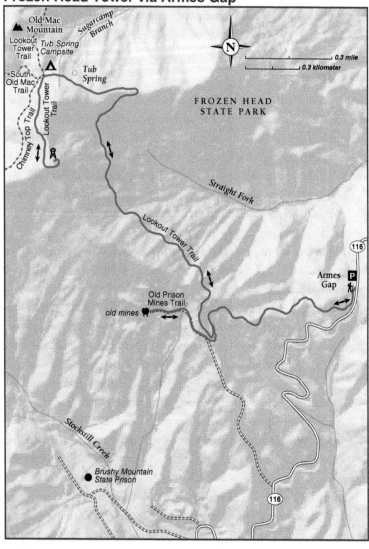

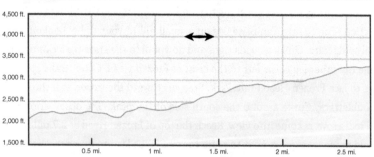

platform built on the infrastructure of a historic fire tower. From the observation platform, you can look west into the valley of Flat Fork and beyond. To the northeast the mountains of Catoosa Wildlife Management Area ripple to the horizon. To the southeast lie Petros, Brushy Mountain Prison, and the Tennessee River Valley. On a clear day the Smoky Mountains are visible and a practiced eye can easily identify the peaks of Mount Le Conte.

From the tower, backtrack 2 miles to the Old Prison Mines Trail. Here, turn right and follow a grassy doubletrack west for a total of 0.4 mile. This old roadbed is much less used than the trail to the tower. Shortly you'll pass by a very small clearing and continue on a level path to enter a more open field after 0.3 mile. Next pass beneath an old stone wall and come to the first mine opening. You can look into the stone maw—through bars—and see the wooden beams that help stabilize the mine. Prisoners from adjacent Brushy Mountain once hand-dug coal beneath Frozen Head, and the mines operated until the 1960s. An old railroad tram led down the mountain to the prison. Imagine the toiling that went on here. Continue beyond this first mine entrance to a couple more openings, bordered by concrete with an old concrete-block guard shack nearby. These were obviously the newer mines. This is your turnaround point. Explore but don't enter the shafts—only a fool enters abandoned mines. Backtrack to the Lookout Tower Trail, returning to Armes Gap for a total hike of 6.2 miles, including the 0.8-mile round-trip segment on the Old Prison Mines Trail.

Nearby Attractions

Frozen Head State Park offers not only hiking but also fishing, camping, and nature study on its 21,000 acres of wildlands. A segment of the Cumberland Trail also travels through the park.

Directions

From Knoxville, take TN 162 (Pellissippi Parkway) toward Oak Ridge, joining TN 62 West to reach Oliver Springs. From Oliver Springs, follow TN 62 West 8.1 miles to TN 116. Look for signs to Petros; then turn right on TN 116 North and travel 4.6 miles, passing through Petros and by Brushy Mountain Prison to Armes Gap. The hike starts on the west side of the gap, to your left, as you drive from Petros.

10 Gallaher Bend Greenway

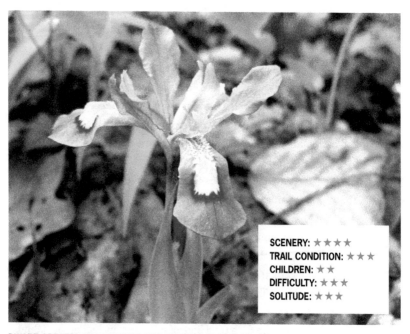

SCENERY: ★ ★ ★ ★
TRAIL CONDITION: ★ ★ ★
CHILDREN: ★ ★
DIFFICULTY: ★ ★ ★
SOLITUDE: ★ ★ ★

DWARF CRESTED IRIS HERALDS THE ARRIVAL OF SPRING.

GPS TRAILHEAD COORDINATES: N35° 57.390' W84° 14.982'

DISTANCE & CONFIGURATION: 4-mile balloon

HIKING TIME: 2.1 hours

HIGHLIGHTS: Lushly wooded trailside, Melton Hill Lake vistas

ELEVATION: 810' at trailhead, 920' at high point

ACCESS: No fees, permits, or passes required; open daily, sunrise–sunset

MAPS: Gallaher Bend Greenway map (tnlandforms.us/greenways/maps03/gb.html),
USGS *Bethel Valley* and *Lovell*

FACILITIES: Restrooms, drinking fountains, swim area, boat ramp at Clark Center Park

WHEELCHAIR ACCESS: Yes, for entire trail

COMMENTS: No pets allowed

CONTACTS: City of Oak Ridge Recreation & Parks Department, 865-425-3450, orrecparks.oakridgetn.gov

Overview

Don't let the moniker *greenway* mislead you. This trek travels through a wooded
wildlife management area on a gravel track deep into a bend on the Clinch River,

here dammed as Melton Hill Lake. Gallaher Bend, located on the Oak Ridge Reservation, is part of the Three Bends, a wildlife preserve of more than 3,000 acres. The trail itself wanders hills and past fields and woods to reach a vista of Melton Hill Lake.

Route Details

This hike will shatter your notions of a greenway—it should be called a trail. After leaving Clark Center Recreation Park, which offers picnicking, boating, and swimming, the trek enters a wildlife management area managed by the Tennessee Wildlife Resources Agency (TWRA). Gallaher Bend is a wildlife-rich area where deer, waterfowl, and game birds enjoy habitat that includes upland woods; fields sown for wildlife; and fields containing native grasses, hedgerows, and miles of shoreline on Melton Hill Lake. This area has remained wild because it is on the Oak Ridge Reservation, land acquired by the U.S. government during the days when Oak Ridge was a secret city working on the atomic bomb that ended World War II. The reservation has been in federal hands for decades, and civilization has sprung up around it, leaving a de facto nature preserve. Today, the area is governed by the U.S. Department of Energy (DOE), but the TWRA does the actual land management. The area is also used for environmental research by the University of Tennessee and the DOE.

On any given day you will find walkers, hikers, and bicyclists traveling from Clark Center Park deep into Gallaher Bend. During the cooler months, the last 0.3 mile of the road leading to the trailhead may be gated, so prepare to add that distance to your hike. Be sure to check the TWRA hunting schedule before you go: tn.gov/twra/hunting/tennessee-hunting-seasons-summary.

The trail starts just beyond the Clark Center Park swimming area on Melton Hill Lake. The gravel doubletrack trail enters a small hollow centered by a creek. Beech, pine, oak, and hickory woods shade the path. Gently climb the first 0.3 mile and open onto a mown field at 0.8 mile. Here, Gallaher Bend is at its narrowest. Melton Hill Lake stretches to the northeast and southwest. The path is bordered by densely growing shortleaf pines, which indicates there was once more field than is visible today. The wide trail allows hikers to walk side by side, and the gravel bed lets you keep your eyes on the scenery rather than watching every footstep.

At 1.1 miles, the trail ascends again. Stone outcrops abut the path as a ridge rises to your left. At 1.4 miles reach a gap and the high point of your hike,

Gallaher Bend Greenway

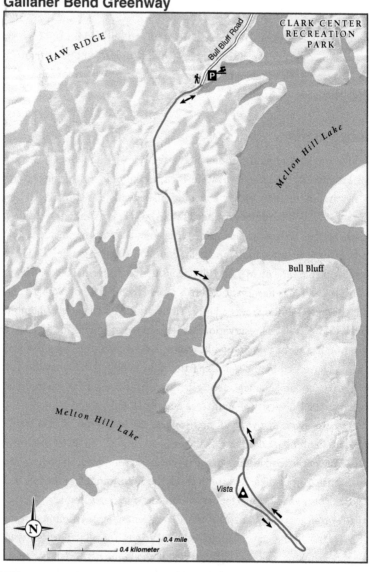

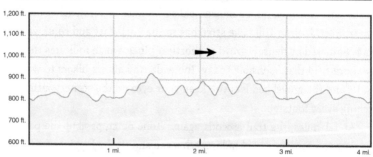

elevationally speaking. The trail levels off, and you reach the loop portion of the trek at 1.6 miles. Here, an old road angles up to the left. This is part of the old Bull Bluff Road that you have been following. The hike, however, stays to the right on the gravel track and shortly opens to a field. Here, you can enjoy eye-popping panoramas down riverine Melton Hill Lake. The Gallaher Bend Greenway makes one last dip before rising to end on a hill at 2 miles. You are nearly at the tip of Gallaher Bend. A gate leads to a field, but our hike joins the primitive track that turns back toward the trailhead. Note the large trees lining the trail. Complete the loop portion of the hike at 2.4 miles. Backtrack 1.6 miles to the trailhead.

Directions

From Knoxville, take TN 162 (Pellissippi Parkway) south toward Oak Ridge, joining TN 62 West. After crossing Melton Hill Lake on a bridge, watch for the Bethel Valley Road exit and join Bethel Valley Road, heading west to reach a traffic light. At the light, turn left on Pumphouse Road where Scarboro Road heads right. Follow Pumphouse Road 0.3 mile, then turn right onto Bull Bluff Road, passing through a gate. At 1.8 miles, reach Clark Center Recreation Park. Continue straight 0.5 mile to reach an outdoor swimming area on your left. Park here. In winter the road will be gated 0.3 mile closer to the entrance of Clark Center Recreation Park.

A COLD-SEASON VIEW ONTO MELTON HILL LAKE

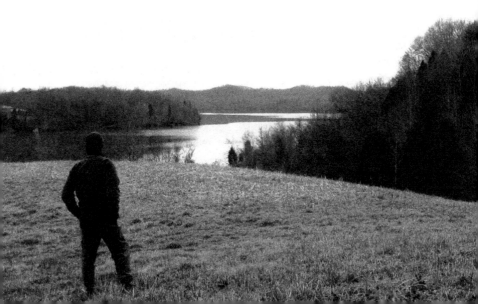

Hall Bend Trail

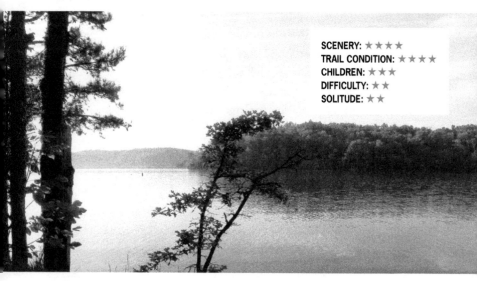

SCENERY: ★ ★ ★ ★
TRAIL CONDITION: ★ ★ ★ ★
CHILDREN: ★ ★ ★
DIFFICULTY: ★ ★
SOLITUDE: ★ ★

THE HALL BEND TRAIL CURVES ALONG SCENIC LAKE COVES LIKE THIS ONE.

GPS TRAILHEAD COORDINATES: N35° 46.462' W84° 15.976'

DISTANCE & CONFIGURATION: 4.5-mile balloon

HIKING TIME: 2.2 hours

OUTSTANDING FEATURES: Lakeside hiking, bluff views, mountain views, good trails

ELEVATION: 820' at trailhead, 950' at high point

ACCESS: No fees, permits, or passes required; open daily, sunrise–sunset

MAPS: Hall Bend Trail map (see website below), USGS *Lenoir City*

FACILITIES: None

WHEELCHAIR ACCESS: None

COMMENTS: None

CONTACTS: Tennessee Valley Authority, 865-632-2101, tva.com/environment/recreation/tva-trails

Overview

Execute a circuit hike along the shores of Tellico Lake at this Tennessee Valley Authority (TVA) Small Wild Area. Start by crossing a flat, then join the winding shoreline with watery views near and far. Make your way to the now dammed Little Tennessee River, where the trail leads to a bluff with spectacular lake, hill, and mountain vistas. Eventually leave the shoreline and return through piney hills, passing a quiet cemetery.

Route Details

Since they began reshaping the Tennessee River Valley nearly a century back, the TVA has flooded prime farmland, drowned quiet communities, and wrought enormous change. But along the way the agency also preserved certain tracts of land—293,000 acres, to be exact—as TVA Small Wild Areas that are kept in their natural state. In the TVA's own words, these areas are "sites with exceptional natural, scenic, or aesthetic qualities that are suitable for low-impact public use, and where some facilities have been installed to help make the land available to the public (e.g., foot trails, signs, parking areas, backcountry campsites)." Other TVA lands are designated Habitat Protection Areas, which shelter threatened or endangered flora and fauna; Ecological Study Areas, containing flora and fauna of scientific interest; and Wildlife Observation Areas, places with concentrated amounts of wildlife.

To allow visitors to explore these areas, the TVA has established more than 170 miles of trails, including the Hall Bend Trail. The well-maintained path hugs the shores of Tellico Lake, then traverses old river bluffs. This bluff climb is but 130 net feet, making this an overall light workout. Cross-trails allow for shortcutting if you don't want to execute the entire loop. The name Hall Bend comes from the last turn of the Little Tennessee River, where it met its mother stream, the Tennessee. Nowadays, the hike is on a remaining neck of land between the two dammed rivers, but the landscape has been drastically altered with the risen waters of Tellico Lake and Fort Loudoun Lake; both dams are within a mile of this hike's trailhead. Tellico Dam stops the Little Tennessee River, while Fort Loudoun Dam backs up the Tennessee River. That's a whole lot of damming going on!

Hall Bend bends no more, but the remaining high ground that is a TVA Small Wild Area allows for quality trekking. Leave the TN 444 trailhead, descending a wide track to a flat saddle dam. What is a saddle dam? Again, in the TVA's words, it is "a non-connecting extension of the main dam that stretches across low spots, raising the surrounding land to an elevation that allows the desired water elevation to be reached. The water elevation in Tellico needed to meet the existing water level in Fort Loudoun [Lake]—the saddle dams allowed this to happen."

This is the first of three saddle dams the hike passes or nears. At 0.3 mile, before you are across Saddle Dam 1, split left as the Hall Bend Trail enters woods and begins running along the shore before returning to the saddle dam at 0.5 mile.

Hall Bend Trail

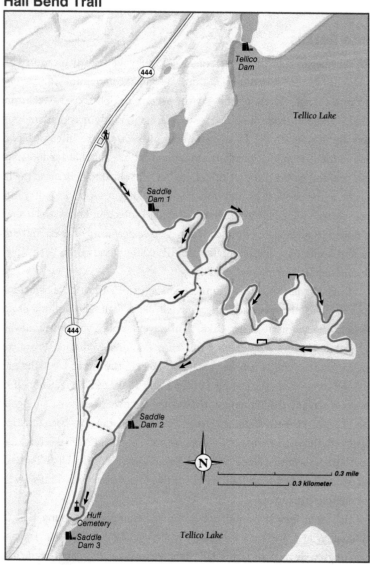

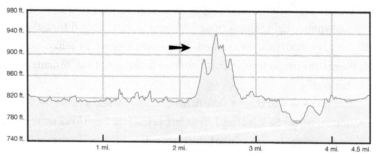

Ahead, come to an intersection and again split left, continuing your shoreline ramble under cover of pine, cedar, hickory, and other hardwoods. Now you begin an extended stretch of staying exactly along or in proximity to the shore.

At 1.1 miles, the first shortcut trail leads you back toward the trailhead; stay with the Hall Bend Trail as it winds generally east in and out of intimate coves. Views of Tellico Dam are common. The singletrack, hiker-only, natural-surface trail reaches the end of the peninsula at 2.1 miles, then joins the old shoreline above the inundated Little Tennessee River channel. Gently rise along a gravelly bluff to reach a view and a bench at 2.3 miles. Majestic mountains rise both east and south above Tellico Lake, and shoreline homes lie across the water. It feels good to be alive and in East Tennessee.

Continue rising along the wooded bluff, where windows in the vegetation allow distant looks and big oaks enhance the forest. Reach a high point at 2.4 miles. By 2.8 miles you are near lake level, and you pass an open area that is Saddle Dam 2. At the dam's south end, a shortcut leaves right, but you keep straight, reentering woods, coming to Saddle Dam 3 at 3.1 miles. Here, the loop turns back north, entering piney forest. TN 444 is through the trees to your left.

Reach the Huff Cemetery at 3.3 miles, just to the right of the trail under trees. The few people interred here were buried a century or more ago, their graves preserved on TVA property. At 3.4 miles, meet the other end of the shortcut you just passed. Keep straight on the natural-surface path, descending to cross a streamlet on a hiker bridge. Ahead, the trail emerges into brushy woods on a sometimes mucky trail. Wind along hills and hollows, tracing an old road part of the way. At 3.9 miles, pop out at Saddle Dam 1. From here, backtrack northwest across the flat to return to the trailhead, completing the trek at 4.5 miles.

Nearby Attractions

Boaters and anglers have three nearby lakes to explore: **Fort Loudoun Lake, Tellico Lake,** and **Watts Bar Lake,** all created by the TVA.

Directions

From Exit 81 off I-75 southwest of Knoxville, take US 321 North—the road actually goes south at this point—for 3.6 miles; then turn right on TN 444 (Tellico Parkway) and follow it 1.6 miles to the Hall Bend trailhead, on your left.

12 Lone Mountain State Forest

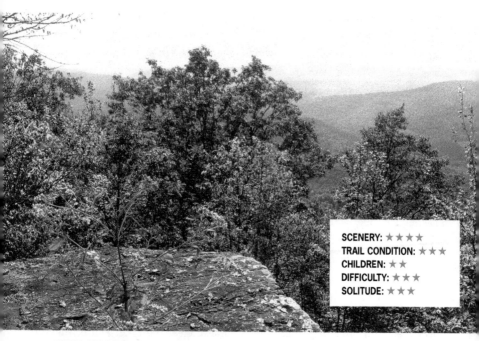

SCENERY: ★ ★ ★ ★
TRAIL CONDITION: ★ ★ ★
CHILDREN: ★ ★
DIFFICULTY: ★ ★ ★
SOLITUDE: ★ ★ ★

YOU'LL BE HOWLING ABOUT THE VIEWS FROM COYOTE POINT.

GPS TRAILHEAD COORDINATES: N36° 04.207' W84° 32.775'

DISTANCE & CONFIGURATION: 7.6-mile out-and-back

HIKING TIME: 4 hours

HIGHLIGHTS: Overlook at Coyote Point, Rankin Spring

ELEVATION: 1,370' at trailhead, 2,200' at high point

ACCESS: No fees, permits, or passes required; open daily, sunrise–sunset

MAPS: Lone Mountain State Forest Recreation Map (see website below), USGS *Camp Austin*

FACILITIES: Picnic table at trailhead, Rankin Spring, and Coyote Point

WHEELCHAIR ACCESS: None

CONTACTS: Lone Mountain State Forest, 865-354-0258, tn.gov/agriculture/forests/state-forests /lone-mountain.html

Overview

Take a trek in a lesser-visited state forest, climbing the slopes of Lone Mountain to reach a rock outcrop and panoramic vista from Coyote Point. The climb is moderate, making it doable by anyone with patience and a decent set of lungs.

Route Details

With approximately 15 miles of trails open to visitors, Lone Mountain State Forest had long been on my hiking radar. And after going there for the first time, I wondered what took me so long to get there. Overshadowed by the nearby and popular Frozen Head State Park, Lone Mountain seems to have been forgotten by many hikers.

Before 1970, Lone Mountain and Frozen Head both were part of the Morgan State Forest. Frozen Head was transferred to the state park system, while Lone Mountain remained part of the state forest. Some tracts of land were acquired by the state in the 1920s from landowner tax default. Another portion was purchased from the Lone Mountain Land Company, which had abused the property. The forest was allowed to regenerate for several decades and is now a scenic destination used by outdoor enthusiasts of all stripes, including hunters. If you are concerned about hiking while the area is being used for hunting, call the forest ahead of time to find out the exact dates.

An archway leads hikers from the trailhead into the state forest. The natural-surface Smokey Bear Trail slices south through oak, holly, and hickory woods. Bridge a tributary of Crooked Fork at 0.2 mile. Shortly, switchback up a ridgeline and then level off. You are expecting the trail to climb, but it doesn't quite yet. You may have to work around occasional muddy areas in the flats. At 1 mile, the trail joins the bulk of the mountain and curves west. Winter views open to the west through the leafless trees. Begin working your way up the east slope of Lone Mountain, entering a steep ravine only to make a sharp switchback to the right at 1.5 miles. The climb eases and partial views open to the east toward Frozen Head.

Swing around to the north side of Lone Mountain, cruising at an elevation of 1,900 feet. Intersect the Longest Mile Trail at 2.1 miles. It continues working westerly along the north slope of Lone Mountain under tulip trees, while the trail to Coyote Point turns left and continues uphill, making a pair of short switchbacks, back in drier forest of black gum and hickory. Pass a small pond to your left at 2.2 miles. By 2.4 miles, you have done nearly all your climbing and are cruising the east slope of Lone Mountain at an elevation of 2,100 feet. The peak of Lone Mountain rises to your right.

At 3.2 miles, reach Rankin Spring, a stone-lined watering hole that is also covered by an open-sided shelter. The water has never looked good here and is not recommended for drinking. However, the area has picnic tables, and there

Lone Mountain State Forest

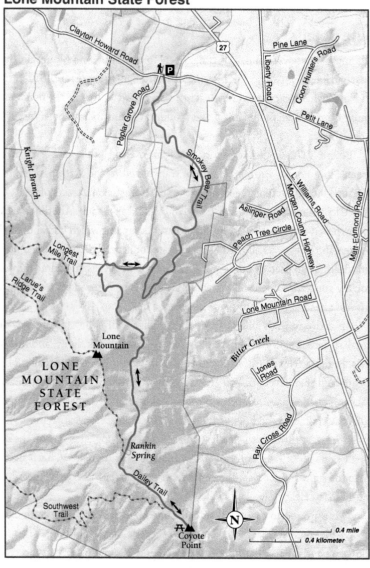

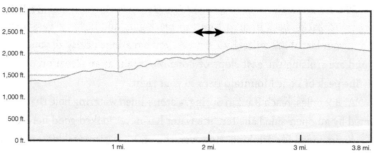

is also a small pond here. It makes a good stopping spot. Just ahead, the Larue's Ridge Trail leaves right and heads over the crest of Lone Mountain. Other area trails are open to hikers and mountain bikers. The Larue's Ridge Trail can be overgrown and is recommended for winter and spring hiking only.

Keep straight here, now on the Dailey Trail. At 3.6 miles, the Southwest Trail leaves to the right for the lower slopes. Continue straight, aiming for Coyote Point. At 3.8 miles, the terrain levels out and you open onto the grass, tree, and rock area of Coyote Point. The rock outcrop extends at the farthest reach of the ridge, allowing you to step out and take in panoramas to the south and west. The cooling towers of Kingston Springs power plant are clearly visible. The bulk of the Cumberland Plateau rises to the west. On a clear winter day you can see the Smokies to the southeast. At this point you're probably wondering, as I was, what took so long to get here. Just be glad you're here, open your pack, and have a relaxing lunch or snack at the picnic tables situated at the overlook.

Nearby Attractions

Frozen Head State Park (see Hikes 8 and 9, pages 54 and 58), just a few miles distant, makes a great camping base from which to explore the 15 miles of trails at Lone Mountain State Forest.

Directions

From Knoxville, take TN 162 (Pellissippi Parkway) toward Oak Ridge, joining TN 62 West to reach Oliver Springs. From Oliver Springs, follow TN 62 West 10.5 miles to Petit Lane. Turn left and follow Petit Lane 1.7 miles to intersect US 27. Cross US 27 and continue straight, now on Clayton Howard Road. Follow Clayton Howard Road 0.4 mile, and reach the trailhead on your left.

13 UT Arboretum Loop

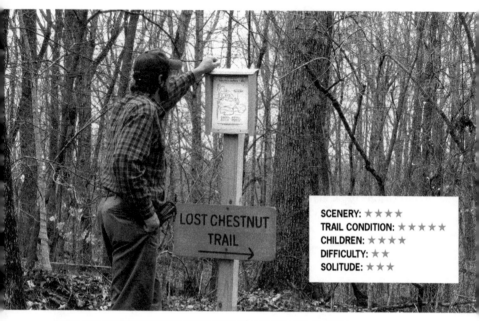

SCENERY: ★ ★ ★ ★
TRAIL CONDITION: ★ ★ ★ ★ ★
CHILDREN: ★ ★ ★ ★
DIFFICULTY: ★ ★
SOLITUDE: ★ ★ ★

MAPS ARE CONVENIENTLY LOCATED AT TRAIL INTERSECTIONS HERE.

GPS TRAILHEAD COORDINATES: N35° 59.620' W84° 13.202'

DISTANCE & CONFIGURATION: 2.3-mile loop

HIKING TIME: 1.2 hours

HIGHLIGHTS: Outdoor education opportunities

ELEVATION: 875' at trailhead, 1,100' at high point

ACCESS: No fees, permits, or passes required; trails open daily, 8 a.m.–sunset

MAPS: UT Arboretum Trail System map (see website below), USGS *Lovell*

FACILITIES: Visitor center with restrooms

WHEELCHAIR ACCESS: None

COMMENTS: No pets or picnicking

CONTACTS: UT Oak Ridge Forest and Arboretum, 865-483-3571, utarboretum.tennessee.edu

Overview

Enjoy a trail network near Oak Ridge at the University of Tennessee Arboretum. Hike interpretive nature trails, learning not only about the trees but also about the ecosystem around you while exploring a variety of environments. Leave the visitor center and explore a hillside before descending to a creek and adjacent wetland. Rise to a high ridge, then work your way down to the trailhead. Allow plenty of time to enjoy the interpretive information.

Route Details

The UT Arboretum is a 250-acre preserve within the greater 2,260-acre Oak Ridge Forest and is headquarters of the University of Tennessee Forest Resources Research and Education Center. The preserve's mission is to establish, collect, and cultivate woody plants, to provide open space for the public to study the forest, and to provide a place to conduct plant-research programs. For the hiker this means a network of interpretive trails lacing the arboretum. Enjoy not only a fine walk in the woods but also an opportunity to absorb interpretive information about our native East Tennessee forests as well as exotic species. The arboretum also has a visitor center that complements the outdoor classroom.

Pick up the Nature Brook Trail near the visitor center, heading southbound. Busy TN 62 hums nearby. Cross a short footbridge and pass through a managed crabapple orchard while scaling a hillside. Enter full-blown woods, passing the Rock Pile Lead Trail. Dip to reach Marsh Road and Scarboro Creek at 0.3 mile. Look for the bald cypresses by the creek. You will also find the central China collection, a group of trees transplanted from that country, where the climate is similar to that of East Tennessee.

Turn left on North Forest Loop Road, then shortly curve right up South Forest Loop Road, and join the Cemetery Ridge Trail within a short distance. The trail system is well marked and maintained, with signs at every junction. Even though some of the trails are labeled as roads, they are used by park personnel only. All pathways are for hikers only. Contemplation benches are scattered throughout the trail system. The gravel Cemetery Ridge Trail climbs away from Scarboro Creek then turns right, passing a sink to meet South Forest Loop Road at 1 mile. Cross Roads Trail is dead ahead. This hike, however, turns right and travels east along South Forest Loop Road. At 1.2 miles, turn right on Backwoods Trail, roaming some of the most remote terrain in the arboretum. Dip to cross an intermittent streambed, then trek through a hickory–oak forest that was a field a century ago. The recuperative powers of nature are on display here.

A final climb leads to yet another trail junction near a TVA power line at 1.5 miles. Pick up the North Forest Loop Road, and then angle away from the

UT Arboretum Loop

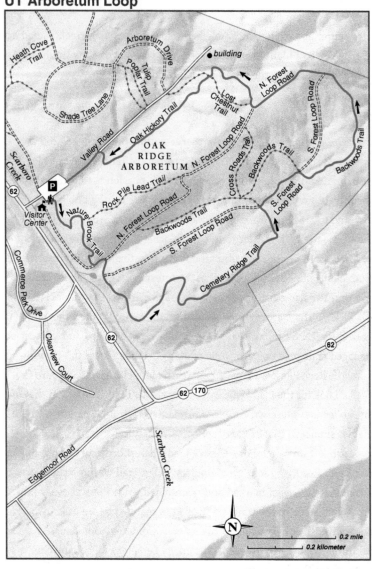

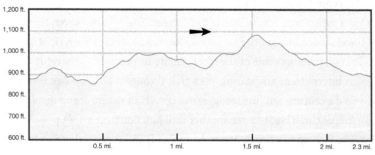

power lines, but not before enjoying a view of the Cumberlands created by the power-line cut.

North Forest Loop Road leads you to another trail intersection at 1.7 miles. Turn right here, joining the Lost Chestnut Trail. Stay right as the Lost Chestnut Trail makes a loop of its own. This trail's name comes from its passing relic stumps from the mighty chestnut tree, which succumbed to blight. Personnel at this forest are involved in developing a strain of blight-resistant chestnuts. At 1.9 miles, look over a display about the chestnut. Keep straight, now on the Oak Hickory Trail, a singletrack path. Note the building below. The UT Arboretum was established in 1964 and currently contains more than 2,500 native and exotic woody plant specimens. Interestingly, UT conducts on-site experiments in plant genetics (such as the one for the chestnut), insects and disease control, and general management of natural resources. This particular hike travels not only by many plant types but also through the associated different habitats. At 2.2 miles, after descending stone and gravel steps, the Oak Hickory Trail reaches Valley Road. Turn left here, continuing downhill to reach the visitor center and complete your hike.

Directions

From Knoxville, take TN 162 (Pellissippi Parkway) toward Oak Ridge, joining TN 62 West (Oak Ridge Highway/South Illinois Avenue). After crossing Melton Hill Lake on a bridge, watch for the Bethel Valley Road exit. Pass the exit for Bethel Valley Road, then look for the signed entrance to the arboretum, about 0.5 mile ahead on your right.

North (Hikes 14–22)

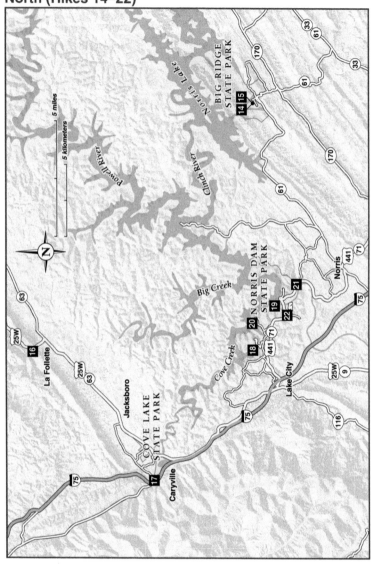

North

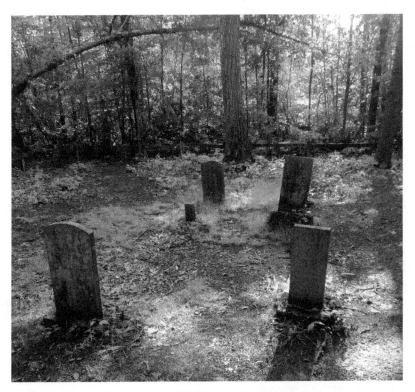

LANGLEY CEMETERY AT BIG RIDGE STATE PARK *(See Hike 15, page 84.)*

14

Big Ridge State Park:
Dark Hollow Loop

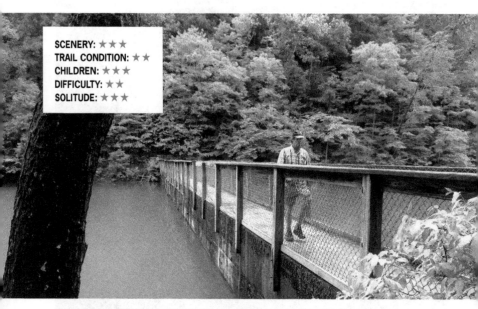

SCENERY: ★ ★ ★
TRAIL CONDITION: ★ ★
CHILDREN: ★ ★ ★
DIFFICULTY: ★ ★
SOLITUDE: ★ ★ ★

A HIKER CROSSES THE DAM DIVIDING BIG RIDGE LAKE FROM NORRIS LAKE.

GPS TRAILHEAD COORDINATES: N36° 14.595' W83° 55.883'

DISTANCE & CONFIGURATION: 5.5-mile balloon

HIKING TIME: 2.8 hours

HIGHLIGHTS: Two lakes, pioneer cemeteries, haunted trail

ELEVATION: 1,030' at trailhead, 1,380' at high point

ACCESS: No fees, permits, or passes required; park open daily, 8 a.m.–sunset

MAPS: Big Ridge State Park map (available at park office, or see website below), USGS *Big Ridge Park* and *White Hollow*

FACILITIES: Restrooms and water fountain at nearby visitor center

WHEELCHAIR ACCESS: None

CONTACTS: Big Ridge State Park, 865-992-5523, tnstateparks.com/parks/big-ridge

Overview

This hike explores the human and natural history of Big Ridge State Park. You first head out from the small park lake, and cross its dam. After traveling the shores of big Norris Lake, you leave the water and enter Dark Hollow, where pioneers toiled. You loop around to pick up Ghost House Trail, where you may have a haunting from one Maston Hutchinson, who is buried in a trailside cemetery. If you make it beyond the cemetery, you'll rejoin the Lake Trail for more watery views. A short backtrack returns you to the trailhead.

Route Details

Big Ridge was one of Tennessee's first state parks. It was developed by the Civilian Conservation Corps (CCC) in conjunction with the building of the Tennessee Valley Authority's first dam, creating Norris Reservoir. The park features rustic CCC stone construction. The lakeside setting of rugged ridge and valley country was once home to simple subsistence farmers. You can still see their homesites, and trails follow wagon roads they used. You can also see their cemeteries, one of which is the resting place of Hutchinson, who is said to haunt the old road/trail that passes near his grave.

Enter the woods, heading north on the singletrack rock-and-dirt Lake Trail. Climb to reach the spur trail to Meditation Point at 0.1 mile. The Lake Trail meanders in mixed woods of pine, hickory, and oak hovering over the slender path, atop a steep ridge dropping off toward the park lake. At 0.4 mile, pass a covered bench. At 0.5 mile, the Loyston Overlook Trail leads left. It climbs 0.3 mile to a knob that offers winter views of Norris Lake. The Lake Trail saddles alongside the park lake, then reaches the dam that separates the park lake from Norris Lake. The park lake is generally kept at the same level, while Norris Lake is raised and lowered under the guidance of the TVA. They factor in flood prevention, energy production, and recreation when they set Norris Lake levels.

Reach the loop portion of the hike at 0.6 mile, heading left on the Dark Hollow Trail into mountain laurel, pine, and cedar. Skirt the shoreline of Norris Lake on a steep slope. What you see is the Bryant Fork arm of the impoundment, and it seriously belies the lake's true size, almost 34,000 acres of water. Circle a small embayment at 0.8 mile, and then turn into Dark Hollow West embayment. Bridge the perennial unnamed stream flowing out of Dark Hollow West at 1.4 miles. Sycamores rise from the streambed. Turn into Dark Hollow to reach the Dark Hollow West backcountry campsite. It is located in a small hollow of Dark Hollow. Join an old wagon track bordered with sweetgum, dogwood, and pine. Look for faint roadbeds, stacked rocks, and other evidence of settlers as you penetrate deeper into the hollow. The path curves above the stream to reach a gap and a four-way trail junction at 2.5 miles.

Big Ridge State Park: Dark Hollow Loop

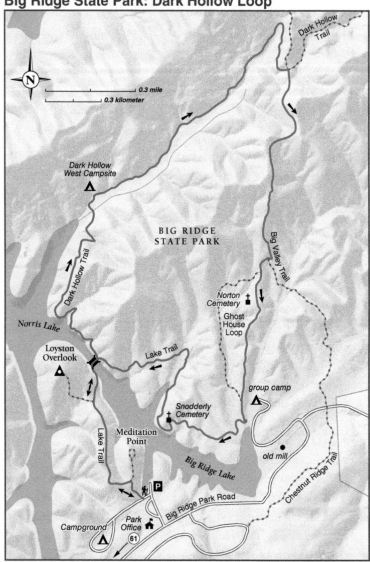

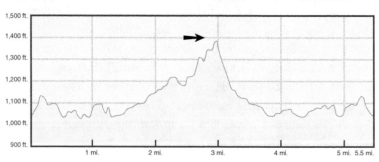

Turn right here, southbound on Big Valley Trail. Follow the old roadbed once used by subsistence farmers to haul corn to the Norton gristmill, located on a spring-fed stream that now feeds the park lake. Pass over Pinnacle Ridge, reaching a high point at 3 miles. Look for beaucoup beech trees up on this ridge, sure evidence that fire suppression has been in place for decades. Under natural, untamed circumstances, this number of beech trees would be found only in the moist hollows.

Descend from the high point to reach a trail junction at 3.2 miles. Head right, joining Ghost House Loop. Hopefully darkness isn't approaching. Just ahead, the trail splits; stay left, still on Ghost House Loop, to reach the Norton Cemetery at 3.4 miles. Find the grave of Hutchinson, who is the spirit responsible for the strange occurrences here and downtrail at his old homesite, now known as the Ghost House. See if you can spot where the home once stood. Be very careful not to stray too far from the marked path.

Meet the other end of Ghost House Loop at 3.7 miles. Keep straight to meet the Lake Trail at 3.8 miles. A spur heads left to the group camp, but this hike turns right, circling the northeast side of the park lake and bridging two streamlets flowing off Pinnacle Ridge. Pass Snodderly Cemetery at 4.2 miles, uphill to your right. The path circles around a tributary, bridging it at 4.5 miles before returning to the park lake. Enjoy some final watery views before finishing the loop portion of the hike at 4.9 miles. Backtrack across the dam to complete the entire 5.5-mile hike. If you have any spare energy, climb to Loyston Overlook, then visit Meditation Point.

Nearby Attractions

Big Ridge State Park also offers fishing, boating, and camping.

Directions

From Knoxville, take TN 33 North to TN 61. Follow TN 61 West 6.3 miles as it winds through hills to reach the state park, on your right. Enter the park and drive a short distance to turn left at the old entrance station. The park office is to your left and offers maps. Continue downhill to park near the lake. The trail starts on the road to the campground.

15

Big Ridge State Park:
Sharps Station Loop

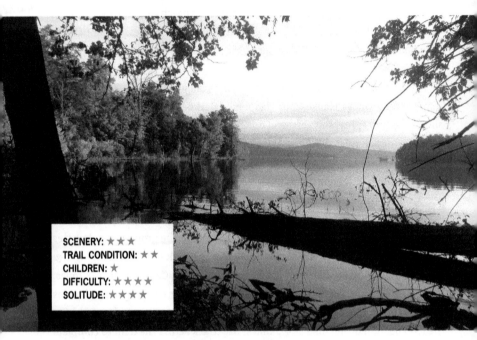

SCENERY: ★ ★ ★
TRAIL CONDITION: ★ ★
CHILDREN: ★
DIFFICULTY: ★ ★ ★ ★
SOLITUDE: ★ ★ ★ ★

LOOKING ONTO NORRIS LAKE FROM THE INDIAN ROCK TRAIL

GPS TRAILHEAD COORDINATES: N36° 14.852' W83° 55.229'

DISTANCE & CONFIGURATION: 6.5-mile balloon

HIKING TIME: 4 hours

HIGHLIGHTS: Norris Lake, pioneer cemetery, historic site

ELEVATION: 1,060' at trailhead, 1,450' at high point

ACCESS: No fees, permits, or passes required; park open daily, 8 a.m.–sunset

MAPS: Big Ridge State Park map (available at park office, or see website below),
USGS *Big Ridge Park* and *White Hollow*

FACILITIES: Restrooms and water fountain at park visitor center

WHEELCHAIR ACCESS: None

COMMENTS: Indian Rock Trail, the loop portion of this hike, can be difficult to follow during the warm season, as it is less used and may be somewhat overgrown. Check with the park office about trail conditions if you are inexperienced.

CONTACTS: Big Ridge State Park, 865-992-5523, tnstateparks.com/parks/big-ridge

Overview

Tread the back reaches of Big Ridge State Park on this trek. Follow old settler roads on the Big Valley Trail, topping Pinnacle Ridge. Pass the Langley Cemetery before scaling Big Ridge. From there, drop steeply to the shores of Norris Lake, where you visit a monument commemorating one of the first settlements west of the Appalachians. Your return route leads steeply up Big Ridge and past Indian Rock, with a winter view. Cruise a high bluff before backtracking to the trailhead.

Route Details

Your destination on this hike—Sharps Station—was one of the first white settlements west of the Appalachian Mountains. What was to be Knoxville, then known as Whites Fort, was the other. Nowadays, Knoxville is a thriving metropolis, while Sharps Station no longer exists. However, a plaque commemorates its location, and you can walk to the site.

Join Big Valley Trail, tracing a roadbed used by pre–Norris Dam settlers as an access to the Norton Gristmill, located near the parking area. Youngish evergreens crowd the trails. Top a hill at 0.3 mile, then dip to a narrow hollow. Bridge a streamlet at 0.5 mile, then climb a gullied track to meet the Ghost House Loop at 0.6 mile. Keep straight on Big Valley Trail, topping Pinnacle Ridge at 0.9 mile. Drift down to meet the Dark Hollow Trail at 1.3 miles.

Leave north from the intersection with the Dark Hollow Trail, climbing from a gap. At 1.6 miles, reach the Langley Cemetery, located on the narrow ridgeline. Most of the graves are simple, unmarked stones. The trail steepens while ascending the south slope of Big Ridge. Top out, catching your breath, then glide downhill, reaching a trail junction at 1.8 miles. Indian Rock Trail, the loop portion of the hike, goes left and right. Stay left, now on a faint singletrack path diving toward Norris Lake, visible through the trees. Watch for paint blazes and flagging tape to help steer your course. The slope eases in mixed woods that were formerly farmland. Turn northeasterly in flats. Step across a stony streambed at 2.2 miles, then turn left along it to meet the lakeshore near an embayment at 2.3 miles. Cruise parallel to the shore, coming to a second embayment. Find a forgotten stone fence, situated along a creekbed, at 2.8 miles. Continue through a cedar grove to reach a trail junction at 3 miles. The next streambed is just ahead. Here, Indian Rock Trail heads right and uphill and is your return route. To reach Sharps Station, stay left on Sharps Station Trail, crossing the

Big Ridge State Park: Sharps Station Loop

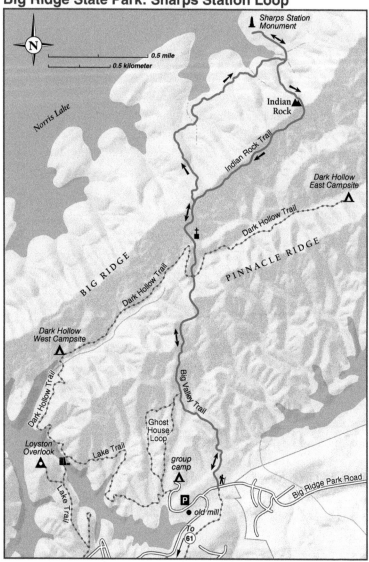

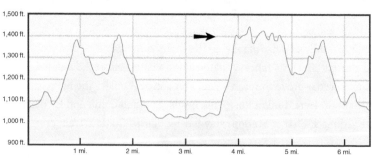

rocky streambed and cruising along a limestone bluff before descending to another streambed. You are in piney flats, keeping the shoreline to your left. The path leads to a lakeside stone marker and nearly obscured gravestones at 3.3 miles. The fort located here provided the settlers protection from Native Americans. The plaque, erected in 1967, mentions a particular December 1794 attack. It is worthwhile to ponder what other events transpired that ultimately led to the abandonment of Sharps Station versus the expansion of Knoxville. Of course, the final blow to Sharps Station was the development of Norris Lake, which led to the displacement of many East Tennessee residents along what was then the free-flowing Clinch River.

Backtrack 0.3 mile from the plaque, enjoying a few lake views. Prepare for a challenging climb up a rib ridge, where you gain nearly 400 feet in 0.3 mile. The ascent eases at an outcrop known as Indian Rock. Here, an early settler named Peter Graves was ambushed and scalped by Native Americans as he was turkey hunting. While following the gobbles of a turkey, he walked right to the natives, who were making the sounds from behind the rock outcrop you see.

The path tops out on Big Ridge, then turns southwest, running along an upturned rock spine shaded by tall trees. Pass a stone fence atop the bluffline at 4 miles, and drop to a gap at 4.2 miles. Undulate along the rocky ridgeline, then complete the loop portion of the hike at 4.7 miles. From here, backtrack 1.8 miles to the trailhead.

Nearby Attractions

Big Ridge State Park also offers fishing, boating, and camping.

Directions

From Knoxville, take TN 33 North to TN 61. Follow TN 61 West 6.3 miles as it winds through hills to reach the state park, on your right. Enter the park and drive a short distance to reach the old entrance station. The park office is to your left and offers maps. Keep straight beyond the station, passing the park cabins. After 0.6 mile reach a stop sign—turn left here, parking near the Norton Gristmill replica. The trailhead is 0.2 mile east from the mill. Backtrack to the stop sign and walk a bit farther to reach Big Valley Trail, on the north side of the road.

16 # Cumberland Trail
Above LaFollette

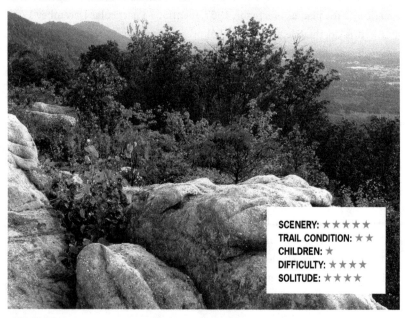

SCENERY: ★ ★ ★ ★ ★
TRAIL CONDITION: ★ ★
CHILDREN: ★
DIFFICULTY: ★ ★ ★
SOLITUDE: ★ ★ ★

THE CUMBERLAND TRAIL IS TENNESSEE'S MASTER PATH.

GPS TRAILHEAD COORDINATES: N36° 23.284' W84° 07.550'

DISTANCE & CONFIGURATION: 5.6-mile out-and-back

HIKING TIME: 3.8 hours

HIGHLIGHTS: Spectacular ridgeline views, knife-edge rocks

ELEVATION: 1,100' at trailhead, 2,000' at high point

ACCESS: No fees, permits, or passes required; open year-round 24/7

MAPS: Cumberland Mountain Segment of the Cumberland Trail (cumberlandtrail.org/trail-segments /cumberland-mountain-segment), USGS *Nydell* and *Jacksboro*

FACILITIES: Trailhead spring

WHEELCHAIR ACCESS: None

COMMENTS: The trail runs through the North Cumberland Wildlife Management Area; you can check for infrequent hunting dates via the Tennessee Wildlife Resources Agency website (tn.gov/twra/hunting). After hiking here, you may want to support Tennessee's master path, the Cumberland Trail. For more information, go to cumberlandtrail.org/get-involved.

CONTACTS: Cumberland Trail Conference, 931-456-6259, cumberlandtrail.org

Overview

This is one spectacular hike. Follow the Cumberland Trail as it leaves the town of LaFollette, then climbs the slope of Cumberland Mountain. You will join a knife-edge ridge with spinelike outcrops that offer expansive vistas. Peer upon LaFollette below, and gaze southward to the Smoky Mountains and westward into the wild Cumberland Plateau, culminating in the Powell Valley Overlook. Beyond this vista, you'll encounter a backcountry trail shelter; a high-elevation stream; and Window Rock, a stone wall with a porthole in it.

Route Details

Big Creek Gap, where this hike begins, is the next major break in Cumberland Mountain south of Cumberland Gap, made famous by Daniel Boone and the Wilderness Road. Thirty miles south of Cumberland Gap, Big Creek Gap made a little history itself. During the Civil War, the gap was much narrower than it is now, before it was widened to allow a road and railway to pass through. Confederate soldiers were stationed above the gap, and it became the site of an 1862 skirmish in which the Confederacy was supplanted from its defensive position by the Union.

Nowadays, Tank Springs, located at the trailhead, attracts locals to the gap. If you hang around long enough, you will see area residents filling jugs and taking the mountain water to their homes for drinking. Cumberland Trail (CT) trekkers can fill their bottles before making the nearly 1,000-foot ascent to the high point of the hike.

Pick up the wide-track path at Tank Springs by walking around a pole gate and passing a trailhead kiosk. Big Creek continues its work, cutting through the gap to your right, and US 25W rumbles with cars and trucks. A railroad line runs to your left. Altogether, you have railroad lines, automobiles, and hikers using the gap, demonstrating its continued importance as a travel corridor.

Big Creek tumbles over rocks large and small, creating rapids and pools. An impressive rock promontory juts forth from the forest across the gap. You will soon be higher than that. But after a half mile, the trail hasn't climbed a bit, and you begin to wonder if you have lost the path, which travels under a railroad trestle spanning Ollis Creek just above its confluence with Big Creek. Beyond the trestle, the Cumberland Trail turns sharply left and begins its ascent of Cumberland Mountain, using multiple switchbacks under a hardwood forest of maple,

Cumberland Trail Above LaFollette

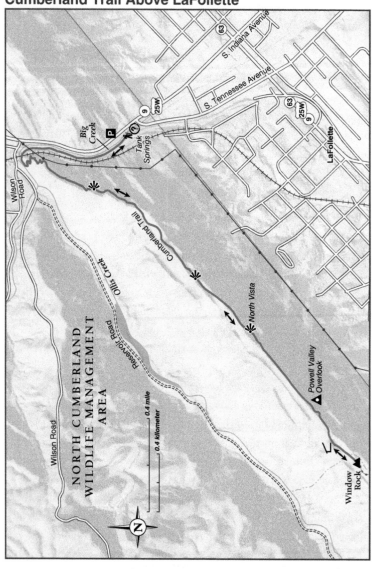

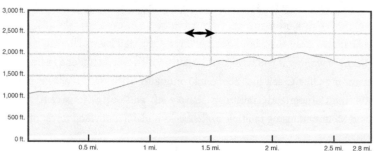

hickory, oak, and magnolia. At 0.7 mile, reach the foundation of a forgotten concrete structure.

Continue climbing as the ridgeline narrows and a rocky spine protrudes
from the soil. Lichens, ferns, and mountain laurel border the path. At 1 mile, the
steep pathway levels off, and you gain obscured views of LaFollette below and
mountains to the north. Serviceberry trees grow among the outcrops. The CT
then curves around the north side of a steep stone promontory, shortly regain-
ing the crest of the ridge. At 1.1 miles, your first unobscured view opens up to
the south, through Big Creek Gap. The crest of Cumberland Mountain briefly
widens, then narrows and becomes rocky again. Keep climbing; you will reach the
1,800-foot elevation mark at 1.3 miles. A brief downgrade is welcome as you slip
around the north side of a rock protrusion to make a shallow gap at 1.5 miles.

The white-blazed CT ascends from the gap on a rock spine, bordered by
pines and mountain laurel, while galax hugs the forest floor. Work your way up
the ragged, jagged crest that resembles upturned shark fins, with a serious drop-
off below. Your next major vista opens at 1.7 miles. Here, LaFollette lies 800
feet beneath you, and the Powell River Valley extends to the east. On a clear day,
Mount Le Conte in the Smokies is easily identifiable. Buzzards may be floating
the nearby thermals.

Dip to another gap at 2 miles, and climb away on another rock spine.
Watch for a vista to the north at 2.1 miles. The contrast is amazing: Cumberland
Mountain divides the civilized Powell River Valley from the scantly populated,
torturous terrain to the north. Reach your high point of 2,000 feet at 2.2 miles.
The trail levels off, and you're walking atop rock slabs bordered by tightly grown
young pine trees.

The views come fast and furious here. Note that the parallel rock ridge to
your right, together with the outcrop you are walking, forms an elevated valley. At 2.6 miles, on a descent, the trail appears to end at an outcrop. You have
reached the Powell Valley Overlook. You can look not only south and east into
the Powell River watershed but also west into the Catoosa Wildlife Management Area, through which the CT travels. Less adventurous hikers may want
to turn around here, but those not afraid of a little rock scrambling on all fours
will work their way down the sandstone ledge (it's not far) before continuing
southwesterly using only leg power to shortly reach a gap. At 2.8 miles, the CT
climbs to a wooden trail shelter and campsite, located in a forested flat beside
rock outcrops. Continue past the shelter and dip to a streamlet cloaked in rhododendron. A rock rampart rises beyond the watercourse. The CT travels along

the rampart in a rich wildflower area. Look for Window Rock, an opening in the rock wall, in this little vale. This is your turnaround point.

Beyond here the CT continues southwesterly atop Cumberland Mountain to reach I-75 and Cove Lake State Park in 9 miles.

Directions

From Knoxville, take I-75 North to Exit 134, for Justin P. Wilson Cumberland Trail State Park. Take US 25W north 8.2 miles to LaFollette and turn left at traffic light #9 (the traffic lights are numbered) onto Indiana Avenue. Follow Indiana Avenue north 0.4 mile to a signed left turn for Justin P. Wilson Cumberland Trail State Park at Tennessee Street, and cross Big Creek. Turn right into a parking area immediately after crossing Big Creek.

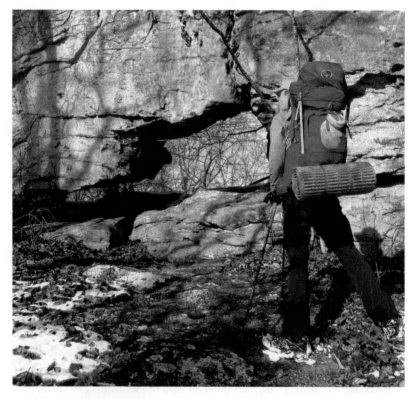

A HIKER ADMIRES WINDOW ROCK.

Devils Racetrack

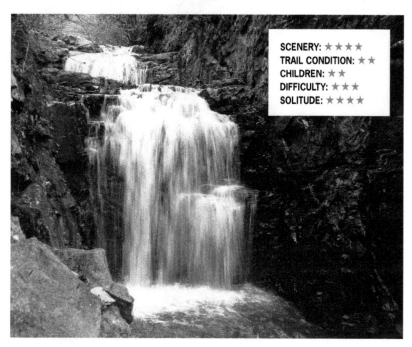

SCENERY: ★ ★ ★ ★
TRAIL CONDITION: ★ ★
CHILDREN: ★ ★
DIFFICULTY: ★ ★ ★
SOLITUDE: ★ ★ ★ ★

BRUCE CREEK FALLS

GPS TRAILHEAD COORDINATES: N36° 18.441' W84° 13.625'

DISTANCE & CONFIGURATION: 6-mile out-and-back

HIKING TIME: 3.4 hours

HIGHLIGHTS: Waterfalls, rock outcrops, wide views

ELEVATION: 1,050' at trailhead, 1,830' at high point

ACCESS: No fees, permits, or passes required; open year-round 24/7

MAPS: Cumberland Mountain Segment of Cumberland Trail (cumberlandtrail.org/trail-segments
/cumberland-mountain-segment), USGS *Jacksboro*

FACILITIES: None

WHEELCHAIR ACCESS: None

CONTACTS: Cumberland Trail Conference, 931-456-6259, cumberlandtrail.org

Overview

This hike uses the Cumberland Trail to (CT) reach a spectacular view from the
rocky western edge of Cumberland Mountain, known as Devils Racetrack. Along

Devils Racetrack

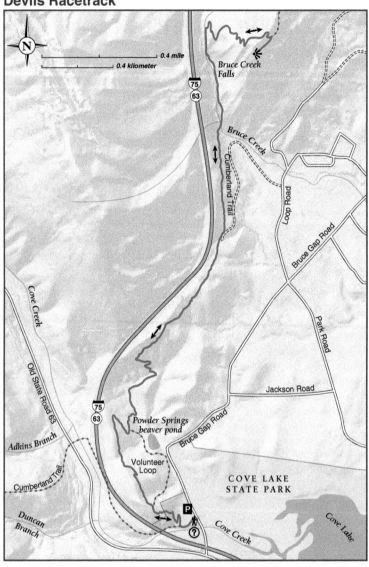

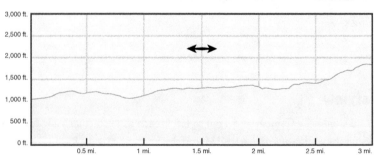

the way you'll pass some steep falls. Be apprised that the trail travels very near I-75, so you will be exposed to road noise. However, the highlights are worth it.

Route Details

Just about everyone who drives north up I-75 from Knoxville notices Devils Racetrack, a series of upturned exposed rock "fins" that rise from the surrounding forest up the crest of Cumberland Mountain. It is only natural that a segment of the Cumberland Trail would travel to this distinct feature. Upon making it to Devils Racetrack, your efforts will be well rewarded with far-reaching views to the south of the Clinch River Valley, much of which is dammed up as Norris Lake. To your west lies an endless series of ridges of the Cumberland Mountains, and you can clearly see the road outline of I-75 as it leads toward Knoxville. Speaking of I-75, it will be your near-constant companion as you travel from the outreaches of Cove Lake State Park north to Devils Racetrack. And yes, it is irritating. That said, I still recommend the hike. Others will second the motion; the trek to Devils Racetrack is increasing in popularity, as is the entire Cumberland Trail.

Leave the Cumberland Trail parking area on a gravel path. Cove Creek flows to your left. Pass a trailside kiosk and keep straight to meet a trail junction. Here, the Smoky Mountain segment of the Cumberland Trail splits left, aiming for Frozen Head State Park. Stay right on a singletrack path that rises by switchbacks. Rich woods with scattered large oaks offer visual beauty. Pass through an old burn with more scrubby woods. After 0.3 mile, reach another trail junction. Here, the Volunteer Loop leads right. You can use it for your return route. The Cumberland Trail keeps its northerly direction. In winter, you will see Cumberland Mountain rising above. Pass a huge oak just before reaching the other end of the Volunteer Loop at 0.8 mile. Descend to a sycamore-laden flat, then ascend along a trickling branch. The CT switchbacks away from the streamlet into a cedar-shaded rock field.

Reach a gap at 1.3 miles. The interstate is just to your left. The CT bridges a giant gully at 1.4 miles, then surmounts a fence at 1.6 miles. You are practically close enough to the interstate to feel a breeze from the trucks going by. Bisect brushy woods that can be overgrown in summer. Views open to the east. Enter a boulder field at 2 miles. This boulder field is clearly not natural. The rocks were sent down the hillside when the interstate was built. The trail opens onto a talus slope, then dips to meet Bruce Creek at an old road at 2.1 miles. Stay left here.

Bruce Creek tumbles in the numerous waterfalls. Yet a closer examination will reveal that the watercourse was rerouted with the building of the interstate. The streambed is not natural, and neither are the falls; the engineers had to work the water down, creating the falls.

Continue through the scenic valley, which shields the road noise. Pass a couple of campsites, reaching Bruce Creek Falls, also known as Triple Falls, at 2.3 miles. Clear water drops in tiers into surprisingly deep pools. At 2.5 miles, bridge Bruce Creek. Begin switchbacking toward the crest of Cumberland Mountain, partially shaded by pines. Briefly level off in a flat before resuming the climb. Pass a huge erratic boulder that tumbled down from the crest of Cumberland Mountain to rest here in the woods. Avoid shortcutting the switchbacks. The building and maintenance of the Cumberland Trail is a mostly volunteer project, so when shortcutting the switchbacks, you cause erosion and mitigate the labor of people who are keeping Tennessee's master path in shape.

The sometimes-sandy trail bed tops out on Cumberland Mountain at 2.9 miles. Turn right here, leaving the CT as it heads northeast to end at Cumberland Gap National Park. Travel a rocky track pocked with low-slung trees. Continue in pure rock to reach the tip of Devils Racetrack at 3 miles. Your trail companion, I-75, is visible below. Southward, you can see Jacksboro in the immediate foreground and greater Knoxville and the crest of the Appalachians in the distance. Easterly, Cumberland Mountain undulates to the horizon. Westerly, the bulk of the Cumberland Plateau rises as a dark, wild rampart. Wow! On your return 3-mile trip, consider taking the Volunteer Loop. It cruises by Powder Springs beaver pond, then meanders low hills before rejoining the CT.

Nearby Attractions

Cove Lake State Park has paved trails, a lake for fishing, and camping.

Directions

From Knoxville, take I-75 North to Exit 134 for Justin P. Wilson Cumberland Trail State Park. After exiting the interstate, turn left, crossing over to the west side of I-75 and away from Cove Lake State Park, on Old Highway 63. Follow Old Highway 63 past the Caryville municipal building for a total of 0.7 mile to Bruce Gap Road. Turn right on Bruce Gap Road and follow it back under the interstate 0.1 mile to the Cumberland Trail parking area on your left.

Norris Dam State Park:
Andrews Ridge Loop

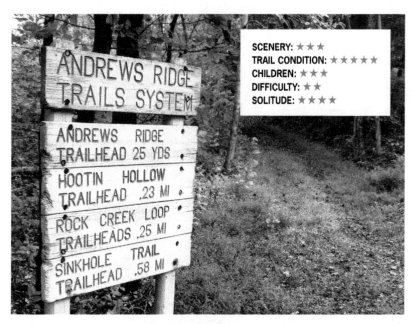

SCENERY: ★ ★ ★	
TRAIL CONDITION: ★ ★ ★ ★ ★	
CHILDREN: ★ ★ ★	
DIFFICULTY: ★ ★	
SOLITUDE: ★ ★ ★ ★	

YOUR GATEWAY TO THE ANDREWS RIDGE TRAILS

GPS TRAILHEAD COORDINATES: N36° 14.506' W84° 07.445'

DISTANCE & CONFIGURATION: 4.7-mile triple loop

HIKING TIME: 2.5 hours

HIGHLIGHTS: Historic homesites, lake views

ELEVATION: 1,340' at trailhead, 1,050' at low point

ACCESS: No fees, permits, or passes required; park open daily, 8 a.m.–sunset

MAPS: Norris Dam State Park Trails map (see website below), USGS *Norris, Lake City, Demory,* and *Jacksboro*

FACILITIES: Restrooms, water at nearby campground

WHEELCHAIR ACCESS: None

CONTACTS: Norris Dam State Park, 865-425-4500, tnstateparks.com/parks/norris-dam

Overview

This hike explores a distinct trail system at Norris Dam State Park. It follows old pioneer roads in hills and hollows homesteaded by rural Tennesseans displaced

Norris Dam State Park: Andrews Ridge Loop

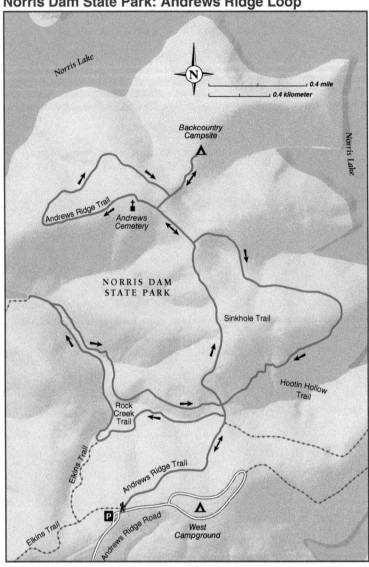

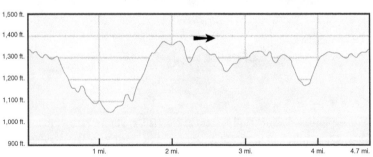

after the development of Norris Lake. Visit a quiet ridgetop cemetery between loops along steeply sloped ground.

Route Details

Andrews Ridge is bordered on three sides by the Cove Creek arm of Norris Lake. The dry hilltop was once home to settlers who labored on its hillsides, scratching out a subsistence living on hardscrabble farms and collecting drinking water from rooftop cisterns. So when word came that the Norris Lake project was going to require them to sell their land, it gave them an opportunity for a new start. Despite the land's less-than-ideal productivity, some people didn't want to move but were forced to. Now Andrews Ridge is part of Norris Dam State Park.

Over the ensuing generations, Andrews Ridge has reverted from field to woodland. The trails you follow trace mostly pioneer roads, weaving around the hills and hollows of the land. I wonder what the former residents would think if they came back to see their land as a recreation destination, with a modern campground and trails.

You start this hike near the West Campground's RV dump station, tracing Andrews Ridge Trail, an old doubletrack road, heading northeast. Here, the Elkins Trail and a connector to the Chuckmore Trail head left, away from our route. Begin to look for artifacts such as old bricks, relics of past settlement. Beech, maple, pine, and tulip trees grow tall on the once-tilled hillsides.

At 0.4 mile, the Hootin Hollow Trail leaves right, curving into an embayment before ending at back at the West Campground. Keep straight on Andrews Ridge Trail and shortly meet Rock Creek Loop. It leads left and downhill, making a loop of its own. Dive into a hollow on Rock Creek Loop. Look for old roads spurring off the main trail, though the way is clear. At 0.6 mile, the Elkins Trail climbs left, but we stay straight to bridge a wet-weather tributary and resume our descent toward Norris Lake. Wooded hills rise sharply around you, cut by streambeds flowing off Andrews Ridge. At 1 mile, reach a junction. Note the old-growth, gray-trunked beech tree here. Continue down the hollow, which is now dominated by sycamores and buckeyes, crossing the main streambed three times to reach the shores of Norris Lake at 1.2 miles. If the water is down, an exposed mud bottom may separate you from the lake. Be careful along the shore or you may find yourself knee-deep in muck. Here, the Elkins Trail heads south to loop back to the trailhead.

Our hike backtracks away from the lake, rising into drier forests of oak and hickory to reach Andrews Ridge at 1.8 miles. Turn left, heading farther north on the Andrews Ridge Trail. Dogwood, black gum, sassafras, and sourwood flank the undulating path. Pass the north end of the Sinkhole Trail at 2.2 miles. At 2.3 miles, reach the loop portion of the Andrews Ridge Trail and stay left, shortly passing the small Andrews Cemetery. Here, lonely graves stand on a high point reclaimed by the forest and creeping periwinkle. Lake views open to the west beyond the cemetery. Meet the spur trail to the park's backcountry campsite at 3.1 miles. Follow it to dead-end at a fire ring and level spot. Overnight hikers must register online or at the park office and bring their own drinking water to this camp. After backtracking from the campsite, complete the loop on Andrews Ridge at 3.4 miles, where you turn left (southeast).

Begin your final circuit at 3.5 miles, turning left on the Sinkhole Trail. This loop curves along the east slope of Andrews Ridge, descending to a gap at 3.6 miles, then resumes following the contours of the lake below. At 4.3 miles, complete the Sinkhole Loop. From here, turn left to backtrack 0.4 mile to the trailhead.

If you want to extend your hike, you can take the Hootin Hollow Trail for 0.7 mile to reach the West Campground and then follow the campground access road to the trailhead.

Nearby Attractions

Norris Dam State Park has recreation opportunities aplenty in addition to trails. Overnight in a cabin, go boating on Norris Lake, or camp in one of two campgrounds to expand your hiking adventure.

Directions

From Exit 128 (Lake City) off I-75, take US 441 South 2.8 miles to the entrance of Norris Dam State Park. Turn left into the entrance, and drive 0.3 mile to a road split. Head left for the West Campground and hiking trails. Drive 1.3 miles to the campground entrance station, across from an RV dump station. There are several parking spots here; please don't block the dump-station road.

19 Norris Dam State Park:
Lake View Trail

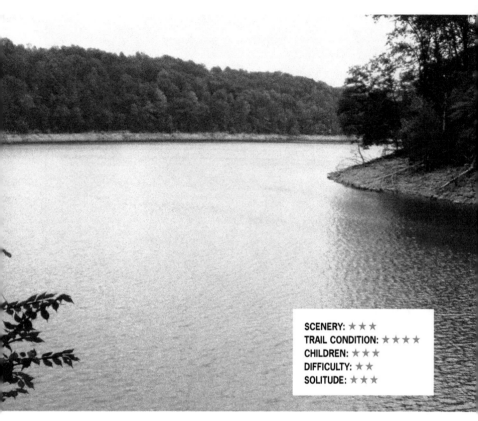

THE RICHLY WOODED SHORELINE OF NORRIS LAKE

SCENERY: ★ ★ ★
TRAIL CONDITION: ★ ★ ★ ★
CHILDREN: ★ ★ ★
DIFFICULTY: ★ ★
SOLITUDE: ★ ★ ★

GPS TRAILHEAD COORDINATES: N36° 13.566' W84° 05.326'

DISTANCE & CONFIGURATION: 3.6-mile triple loop

HIKING TIME: 2 hours

HIGHLIGHTS: Lake views, big trees

ELEVATION: 1,070' at trailhead, 1,450' at high point

ACCESS: No fees, passes, or permits required; park open daily, 8 a.m.–sunset

MAPS: Norris Dam State Park Trails map (see website below), USGS *Norris*

FACILITIES: Restrooms, water, and picnic area at state park and nearby dam visitor center

WHEELCHAIR ACCESS: None

CONTACTS: Norris Dam State Park, 865-425-4500, tnstateparks.com/parks/norris-dam

Norris Dam State Park: Lake View Trail

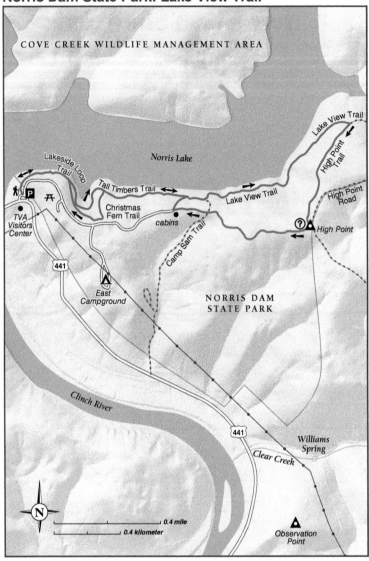

COVE CREEK WILDLIFE MANAGEMENT AREA

Norris Lake

Lakeside Loop Trail

Tall Timbers Trail

Lake View Trail

High Point Trail

Christmas Fern Trail

cabins

Camp Sam Trail

TVA Visitors Center

441

High Point Road

High Point

East Campground

NORRIS DAM STATE PARK

Clinch River

441

Williams Spring

Clear Creek

N

0.4 mile
0.4 kilometer

Observation Point

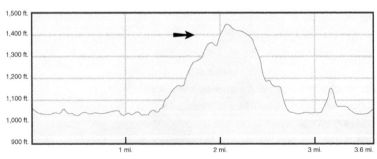

Overview

Norris Dam State Park was originally developed in the 1930s. Over nine decades it has undergone many changes and displayed several recreational faces for visitors. This hike wanders a north-facing slope overlooking the lowermost part of Norris Lake, near Norris Dam, on a Civilian Conservation Corps–built track, traveling a steep slope with views of many big trees along the way. You then pick up the Lake View Trail, which explores more shoreline, with expansive water vistas, everywhere-you-look beauty, and still more big trees. Pass High Point on the return trip before joining nature trails that return you to Norris Dam. You will have to negotiate many trail junctions, but the way is clear and navigable by anyone.

Route Details

The trek begins on a hiker-only asphalt path, Lakeside Loop Trail, leaving from big Norris Dam. Rich woods of beech tower overhead as you travel the hillside, roughly paralleling the shoreline. The trail shortly changes to gravel. An angler's trail spurs left toward the shore, while the main track makes an easterly course under shade-bearing beech trees. The still waters of Norris Lake are visible through the trees no matter the season. After a quarter mile the trail splits. Take the left fork, staying closer to the lake. At 0.3 mile, some old steps lead down to the lake, from an earlier recreational incarnation of the park. These seem like part of an old dock. The first of many clear lake views opens at this locale.

Continue on the moist north slope and shortly reach another junction. Here, Christmas Fern Trail leads right and uphill, but you stay left, joining Tall Timbers Trail. Begin curving around a cove of the lake under sycamore and tulip trees, making a mostly level track. Benches are set along the path, should you choose to relax. Meet the other end of Christmas Fern Trail at 0.5 mile. Keep straight on Tall Timbers Trail, still within the original state park trail system, built so long ago.

At 0.9 mile, you leave the older trail system and join the multiuse Lake View Trail. This path ties together trails of the state park along with those of the City of Norris Watershed, though Lake View Trail stays within the bounds of the state park. Pass a horse barrier, then reach yet another split. Stay left as a sign warns equestrians to walk their horses on the supersteep gravelly track. Lunge toward Norris Lake.

Continue easterly in oak woods, also looking for impressively sized buckeye and beech trees, including a huge old-growth beech at 1.3 miles on trail right. You'll experience more vertical variation in this section. Cove Creek Wildlife Management Area stands across the lake and provides a natural shoreline vista across the dammed waters of the Clinch River.

At 1.6 miles, meet the High Point Spur, which cuts back acutely right and uphill. Take this trail as it climbs through huge oak trees to reach High Point, a wooded spot (no views) at a trail intersection, at 2.1 miles. You are nearly 400 feet higher than when you started. A trailside kiosk helps keep hikers oriented. Turn right here, now heading west on a doubletrack trail. Short spurs dead-end; just stay with the well-trod path.

At 2.3 miles, the path angles right and downhill, passing around a chain-link gate. Keep descending under more big oaks to reach a four-way trail junction at 2.5 miles. Here, the Camp Sam Trail leads left and a spur trail leads right, back toward the Lake View Trail. This hike keeps forward to pass around a gate and reach a park cabin cluster. Pass Cabin #10 on your left, then look for a slender trail leading right, away from the cabins, at 2.6 miles; take this trail to return to the Tall Timbers Trail.

Begin backtracking at 2.7 miles, again in the network of old nature trails, heading left (west) along Tall Timbers Trail. Enjoy some new terrain as you pick up the Christmas Fern Trail leading left and uphill at 3.1 miles. Ascend through paw-paws, nearing a park road before dropping to another intersection at 3.3 miles. Keep left on the Lakeview Loop Trail to return to the trailhead.

Nearby Attractions

Norris Dam State Park has recreational opportunities aplenty in addition to trails. Overnight in a cabin, go boating on Norris Lake, or camp in one of two campgrounds to expand your hiking adventure.

Directions

From Knoxville, take I-75 North to Exit 122. Turn right on TN 61 East, and follow it 1.4 miles to US 441. Turn left and take US 441 North 4.9 miles, passing the TVA visitor center on your left just before you reach Norris Dam State Park's East Area. Park in the circular lot on the right, just before US 441 crosses Norris Dam.

20 # Norris Dam State Park:
Marine Railway Loop

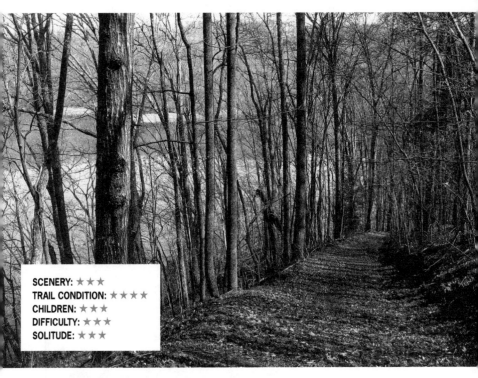

WINTER VIEW OF NORRIS LAKE FROM THE TRAIL

SCENERY: ★ ★ ★
TRAIL CONDITION: ★ ★ ★ ★
CHILDREN: ★ ★ ★
DIFFICULTY: ★ ★ ★
SOLITUDE: ★ ★ ★

GPS TRAILHEAD COORDINATES: N36° 14.598' W84° 06.132'

DISTANCE & CONFIGURATION: 3.5-mile double loop

HIKING TIME: 2 hours

HIGHLIGHTS: Lake views, wide trail

ELEVATION: 1,310' at trailhead, 1,050' at low point

ACCESS: No fees, permits, or passes required; park open daily, 8 a.m.–sunset

MAPS: Norris Dam State Park Trails map (see website below), USGS *Norris*

FACILITIES: Restrooms, water, picnic tables, playground, campground at state park

WHEELCHAIR ACCESS: None

COMMENTS: Cabins at trailhead

CONTACTS: Norris Dam State Park, 865-425-4500, tnstateparks.com/parks/norris-dam

Norris Dam State Park: Marine Railway Loop

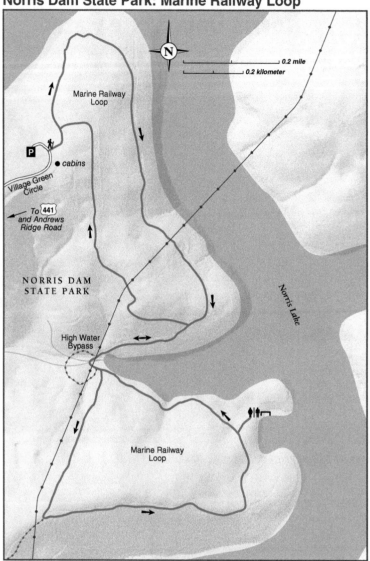

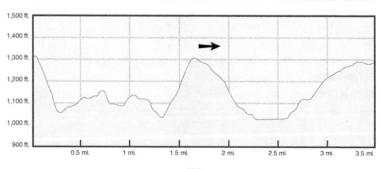

Overview

This doubletrack path starts atop a knobby ridge before plunging toward Norris Lake, where it travels near the shore through second-growth forest. The hike then turns up an inlet, where it makes a second loop and climbs the knobby ridge again, only to return to Norris Lake, this time passing directly along accessible shoreline. Your second climb, back to the trailhead, is gentler.

Route Details

Norris Dam State Park is chock-full of trails. The Marine Railway Loop is but one hiking opportunity, but trail treaders seem to gravitate to this path because so much of it goes along scenic Norris Lake. What started as a flood-control project (Norris Dam) begun during the Great Depression has resulted in this park with lake, river, and land recreation administered by the State of Tennessee and the Tennessee Valley Authority, commonly referred to as the TVA and headquartered in Knoxville.

The hike makes somewhat of an odd start, as you have to walk behind Cabin #8, a state park rental cabin that may be occupied. But don't sweat it; pick up the wide trail leading downhill and left away from Cabin #8. Shortly reach a signed trail intersection and the beginning of the actual Marine Railway Loop. Turn left (north), heading sharply downhill on a shaded doubletrack path that makes walking easy and allows you to enjoy the surrounding woodland environs. In winter you will already be viewing Norris Lake as it nearly encircles the peninsula down which you hike.

Chestnut oak, red oak, maple, and other hardwoods shade the path as it dives for the water. Norris Lake is quite serpentine. The dammed waters of the Clinch and Powell Rivers both cut torturous courses through the knobby ridges forming the transition between the Cumberland Plateau and the Tennessee River Valley. It is this relationship between water and land that makes Norris Lake one of the most scenic bodies of water in the South.

Level off after 0.25 mile, then curve east. The impoundment, with all its fingerlike inlets, lies to your left. You are actually on the Cove Creek Arm of the lake. Red maple, tulip, dogwood, and beech trees find their niche in the forest, while pine, cedar, and the occasional hemlock add year-round greenery. Pass under a power-line cut at 0.8 mile. Of course, having a power line so near the electricity-generating Norris Dam should be no surprise. The clear-cut offers an unobstructed vantage of Norris Lake. At 0.9 mile, turn into a narrow bay. Reach a trail junction at 1 mile. Your return route and the first loop leave to the right, but you stay left, heading for the second loop along the narrow bay.

The trail descends toward the top of the inlet. Watch as the High Water Bypass leaves to the right. Use the bypass when Norris Lake is up and floods the main trail; otherwise, curve around the inlet, ignoring a closed power-line access road at the inlet head. Reach a trail junction at 1.3 miles. Here, the other end of the High Water Bypass enters, and just ahead the second loop begins. Turn right here (south), aiming up the hill under the power line. It's an ugly, steep climb, and you can see every bit of elevation to be gained. Numerically speaking, it is 280 feet in 0.3 mile, where you reach a trail junction. The trail leading right, still southerly, meets US 441 and is an alternate trailhead for the Marine Railway Loop. This hike, however, leads acutely left, east, toward Norris Lake.

The downgrade is shaded by hardwoods and is gentler than the climb you just made, descending the same distance climbed in 0.5 mile. Norris Dam is visible through the trees to the south. Drift into flatlands and reach a trail junction at 2.2 miles. Here, a spur trail leaves right to a bench overlooking a piney peninsula and a lake-access point where you could swim or play fetch with a water-loving dog. When the lake is at its drawn-down winter levels, you will see artificial fish-attraction structures embedded in the lake bottom.

Resume the loop, again curving along the inlet, this time directly along the shoreline. Note the numerous trees fallen into the lake's edge. They also provide good fish habitat. Reach a trail junction at 2.5 miles, completing the second loop. Backtrack around the inlet and reach the first loop at 2.8 miles. Stay left (northwest), making your second climb, which is fairly gradual. Pass under the power line a final time. Resume hiking under hardwoods, watching for redbuds and dogwoods. As you complete the second loop, Cabin #8 is within sight through the trees. Backtrack to the trailhead to complete the 3.5-mile hike.

Nearby Attractions

Norris Dam State Park has recreational opportunities aplenty in addition to trails. Overnight in a cabin, go boating on Norris Lake, or camp in one of two campgrounds to expand your hiking adventure.

Other trails are nearby. The **Andrews Ridge trail system** is detailed in this guidebook on page 97. It leaves from the state park's West Campground. The **Norris Watershed Trails,** also known as the East Park Trail System, explores the terrain east of Norris Dam. The TVA offers still more trails, including **River Bluff Trail**, detailed in this book on page 114.

Directions

From Exit 128 (Lake City) off I-75, take US 441 South 2.8 miles to the entrance of Norris Dam State Park. Turn left to enter the park, and drive 0.3 mile to a road split; stay right, heading toward the park office and park cabins. Stop at the park office on your left to get a trail map, then continue toward the cabins, following the paved road to its end in a cul-de-sac. Park here. To pick up the trail, walk a short distance back toward Cabin #8; the trail starts behind the cabin.

LOOKING DOWN ON A QUIET COVE OF NORRIS LAKE

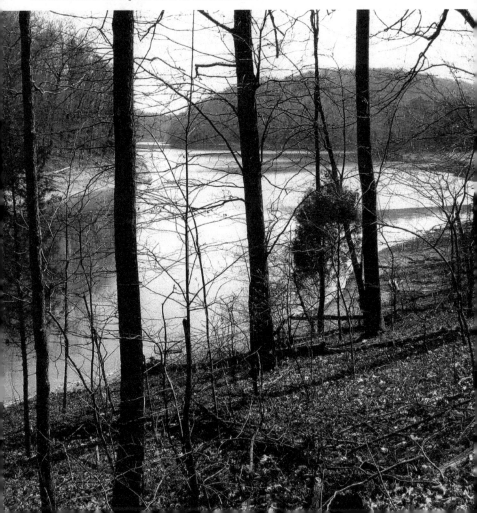

Observation Point Loop

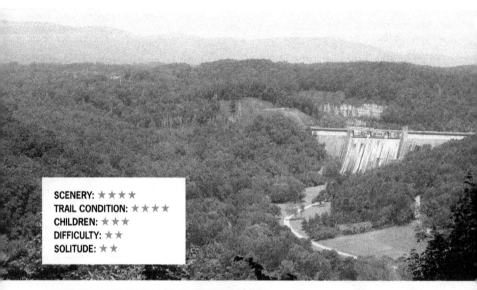

SCENERY: ★ ★ ★ ★
TRAIL CONDITION: ★ ★ ★ ★
CHILDREN: ★ ★ ★
DIFFICULTY: ★ ★
SOLITUDE: ★ ★

NORRIS DAM AS SEEN FROM OBSERVATION POINT

GPS TRAILHEAD COORDINATES: N36° 12.783' W84° 04.347'

DISTANCE & CONFIGURATION: 3.7-mile loop

HIKING TIME: 2 hours

HIGHLIGHTS: Historic gristmill, cleared vistas

ELEVATION: 880' at trailhead, 1,360' at high point

ACCESS: No fees, permits, or passes required; open daily, sunrise–sunset

MAPS: Norris Watershed Trail Map (cityofnorris.com/id336.html), USGS *Norris*

FACILITIES: Restrooms, water fountain, picnic tables at Norris Dam visitor center

WHEELCHAIR ACCESS: None

COMMENTS: This is but one hike in the extensive Norris Watershed trail system.

CONTACTS: City of Norris, 865-494-7645, cityofnorris.com

Overview

This is a great hike on land originally acquired by the TVA as part of Norris Dam, on trails developed by the Civilian Conservation Corps in the 1930s. Begin on scenic Clear Creek at a historic gristmill. Travel along the cool valley of the stream before rising to a view atop Reservoir Hill. Travel through tall timber to Observation Point, a superlative clear overlook of the Clinch River Valley,

Norris Dam, and Cumberland Mountain beyond. Descend along a steep riverside bluff to complete the loop.

Route Details

The Norris Watershed trails are located below Norris Dam. They offer well-marked and maintained singletrack and doubletrack paths winding through a surprisingly large area, especially when combined with the property of adjacent Norris Dam State Park. This particular hike travels along lower Clear Creek, a slender, crystalline stream broken by small dams. The path then leaves the stream and ascends into hickories and oaks on Reservoir Hill, site of a large water-storage tank and a shaded picnic area with attractive stonework. Travel under some large trees that perhaps escaped the logger's ax before making a side trip to aptly named Observation Point, an overlook that accurately captures East Tennessee with its rivers, ridges, mountains, and lakes. It also captures the essence of the Tennessee Valley Authority (TVA), which shaped this land and its people as much as any other single influence.

The hike begins at the old gristmill (see photo on page 201). Explore the primitive power plant, parts of which have been in operation since 1798. The mill, originally built in nearby Union County, Tennessee, has undergone many changes and was moved to its present site; otherwise, it would have been flooded under Norris Lake, as so many other relics of pre-TVA days were. Follow Clear Creek Trail beyond the mill, joining a sluiceway that delivers water from Williams Spring to turn the mill wheel. Pass the springhead, emerging from the base of a tree. Travel under a pair of power-line cuts, as a spur path goes to a streamside picnic area. Meet Dyer Hollow Trail at 0.3 mile. Keep straight on Clear Creek Trail, curving past some small stone dams over which the stream spills noisily. This was once the site of a now-vanished gristmill.

The cool, moist corridor is good for spring wildflowers. Reach Lower Clear Creek Road at 0.7 mile. Look across the road for the rectangular water runs from a small fish hatchery. Interestingly, the TVA wasn't sure if fish would reproduce in an impoundment such as Norris Lake; thus they built several fish hatcheries to stock the impoundment. (For the record, fish do reproduce in Norris Lake; ask any local angler.) Clear Creek Trail now wanders the far side of Clear Creek. You can take it or walk up the road to the Norris water treatment plant. Here, Hi Point Trail leaves left as a road across Clear Creek. Stay right, joining Reservoir Hill Trail as it turns south and runs parallel to Lower Clear Creek Road.

Observation Point Loop

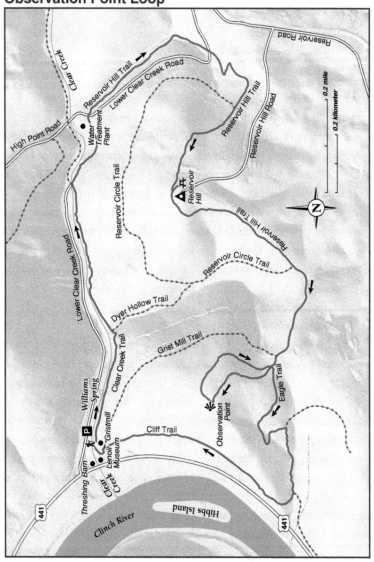

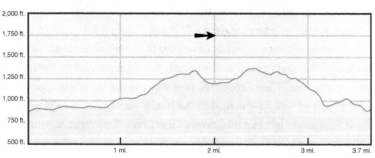

Ascend, crossing Lower Clear Creek Road at 1.2 miles. Keep climbing into oaks, passing a sinkhole before meeting Reservoir Circle Trail at 1.4 miles. After more climbing, you'll come to a decorative stone wall and shaded picnic area at 1.7 miles. Spur trails lead to the picnic area, where you can grab a view through the trees of Norris Dam. Head downhill among large, regal oaks. Intersect the other end of Reservoir Circle Trail at 2 miles. Keep straight, bisecting two power-line clearings before meeting the Grist Mill Trail at 2.3 miles. It's just 0.7 mile to the parking area, but why cut the hike short when the best is yet to come?

Instead, keep straight, and in a few feet arrive at another junction. Here, take the teardrop-shaped Observation Point Trail. Loop up to a gazebo and Observation Point at 2.5 miles. Here, you can gaze northwest to soak in Norris Dam, the Clinch River flowing below, hills spreading off, and finally Cumberland Mountain rising in the background. What a sight! No wonder the CCC routed a trail here! Listen to the roar as the Clinch flows over the weir dam below.

Loop back down to the junction, then pick up the Eagle Trail, a slender singletrack path descending west off the hill of Observation Point. Pass a dead-end trail leaving left at 3 miles, then continue descending a hollow to reach another intersection at 3.1 miles. A spur leads left down to US 441. Watch for a low-flow fall dripping over a stone lip just above this junction. Our hike leaves right and uphill on the Cliff Trail. Curve onto a sharply sloped wooded bluff above the Clinch River. Look down on the river and weir dam. The slope eases and you meet the Grist Mill Trail just before coming to the W. G. Lenoir Museum. It is but a short walk to the trailhead from the museum.

Nearby Attractions

Norris Dam State Park (see previous three hikes) offers camping, picnicking, and more hiking. The **Clinch River** has first-rate trout fishing and paddling opportunities. Norris Lake offers flatwater boating and fishing.

Directions

From Knoxville, take I-75 North to Exit 122. Turn right on TN 61 East and follow it 1.4 miles to US 441. Turn left on US 441 North; after 3.6 miles, just past the W. G. Lenoir Museum, look for the right turn to Lower Clear Creek Road and a sign for the old gristmill. Park by the gristmill. If this lot is full, park at the Lenoir Museum (2121 Norris Freeway).

22 **River Bluff Trail**

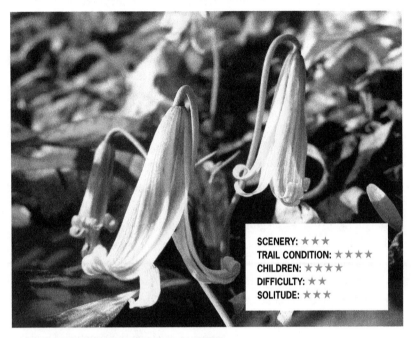

SCENERY: ★ ★ ★
TRAIL CONDITION: ★ ★ ★ ★
CHILDREN: ★ ★ ★ ★
DIFFICULTY: ★ ★
SOLITUDE: ★ ★ ★

WILDFLOWERS ABOUND ON THIS TRAIL IN SPRING.

GPS TRAILHEAD COORDINATES: N36° 13.227' W84° 05.703'

DISTANCE & CONFIGURATION: 3.3-mile loop

HIKING TIME: 1.9 hours

HIGHLIGHTS: River views, spring wildflowers

ELEVATION: 820' at low point, 1,140' at high point

ACCESS: No fees, permits, or passes required; open daily, 8 a.m.–sunset

MAPS: River Bluff Trail map (see website below), Norris Dam State Park map (tnstateparks.com/parks
/norris-dam), USGS *Norris*

FACILITIES: None

WHEELCHAIR ACCESS: None

COMMENTS: Many other trails are located nearby on this TVA property and at Norris Dam State Park.

CONTACTS: Tennessee Valley Authority, 865-632-2101, tva.com/environment/recreation/tva-trails

Overview

The Tennessee Valley Authority (TVA) did a good job in locating a trail on this
bluff below Norris Dam. The steep, north-facing slope overlooks the Clinch

River and offers superlative wildflower displays amid sheer rock outcrops and tall forest. It also provides a good workout when the path climbs the bluff after traveling downstream along the trout-filled tailwater. The return trip meanders under oaks along the bluff edge, exploring multiple environments.

Route Details

Leave easterly from the parking area on a singletrack footpath. The federally designated National Recreation Trail travels beneath white oak, hickory, beech, and holly in a TVA-designated natural area. The moist, north-facing slope upon which it travels makes it nearly ideal for wildflowers in April. Among the spring offerings you will see are trillium, trout lily, mayapple, toothwort, and wild ginger. The path drifts closer to the Clinch River, which Norris Dam impounds as Norris Lake. The dam is located within sight of the trail. In winter you can easily see the concrete behemoth through the trees. On a still day you will undoubtedly hear the hum of the dam as its turbines create electricity.

Norris Dam was the TVA's first impoundment, completed in 1936. Many residents were unhappy about being removed from the fertile riverside lands for Norris Lake. The TVA tried to make good relations by showing how the project would benefit the greater whole of society. One way they did this was making demonstration parks along the newly created lake and dam. The lands that the River Bluff Trail explores are part of the demonstration parks, as are nearby Norris Dam State Park and Big Ridge State Park, both of which feature hiking trails included in this guidebook.

Reach the loop portion of your hike at 0.3 mile. Stay left, still easterly, on the singletrack. Ferns and mosses also thrive on this north slope. Bridge a steep, wet-weather stream at 0.4 mile. Trout lilies seemingly cover the entire slope in this area during April. Come along the Clinch River at 0.7 mile. The clear, aqua water is quite cold after emerging from the dam base. This icy water supports a renowned trout fishery. In summer you may feel a cool breeze blowing off the water. Depending upon whether the dam is generating, you may see anglers in waders or in boats fishing the river. Fallen trees line the water's edge and provide habitat for trout. On the land, mossy rock outcrops rise above you. Buckeye trees are quite common on this lower slope.

Thus far the elevation undulations have been negligible. Look uphill for a sheer bluff rising forth from the thick forest. The trail traces the river as the waterway turns southeasterly. At 1.4 miles, watch for a boat ramp across the

River Bluff Trail

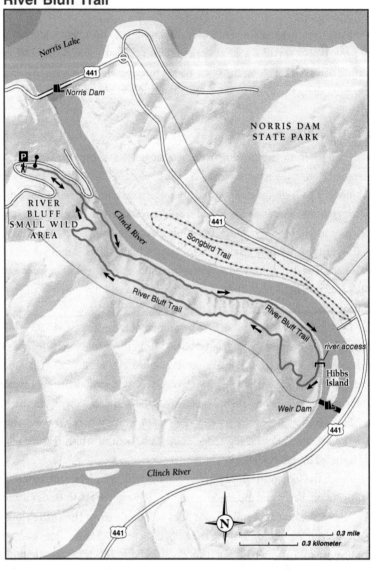

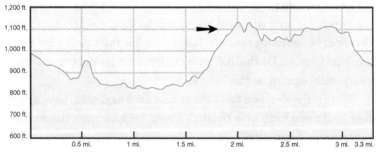

river, as well as trails. In winter you may even see hikers walking the Songbird Trail, an easy loop trek on level terrain, also across the river. At 1.5 miles, come to a bench and a trail leading left to river access. Walk down and touch the chilly water as it divides around the head of Hibbs Island. A weir dam located at the base of Hibbs Island oxygenates the water, making it a better environment for fish and other aquatic species.

The River Bluff Trail turns away from the water, making a pair of switchbacks as it heads for higher ground. The Clinch continues its journey, only to be impounded by Melton Hill Reservoir, then freed once again to meet the Tennessee River near the town of Kingston. Rise into oak-dominated woods, huffing and puffing your way to reach a high point at 1.8 miles. Congratulations! You just climbed nearly 300 feet. Join the upper end of the bluff, heading west. The Clinch looks much smaller from up here. Watch for some sizable oaks and creamy-white dogwood blossoms in spring. Wintertime views open on the dam and Norris Lake to the north.

At 2.3 miles, come near a closed forest road in a gap. Continue your wooded forest walk. At 2.7 miles, the slender River Bluff Trail switchbacks sharply downhill. A second switchback hastens the descent, and at 3 miles you find yourself completing the loop portion of the hike. Backtrack 0.3 mile to the trailhead.

Nearby Attractions

Norris Dam and **Norris Dam State Park** (see Hikes 18–20) are a stone's throw from this trail. Paddlers and anglers will be interested in plying the Clinch River, with its nationally recognized tailwater trout fishery. The chilly Clinch makes a fun float for nonanglers as well, when Norris Dam is generating.

Directions

From Exit 128 (Lake City) off I-75 north of Knoxville, take US 441 South for 3.8 miles; then turn right on Dabney Lane, which is before Norris Dam but after Norris Dam State Park. Follow Dabney Lane just a few feet, then veer left on a paved road heading downhill, with a sign indicating NORRIS DAM. Follow the paved road 0.7 mile to end at a gate and the trailhead for the River Bluff Trail.

East (Hikes 23–27)

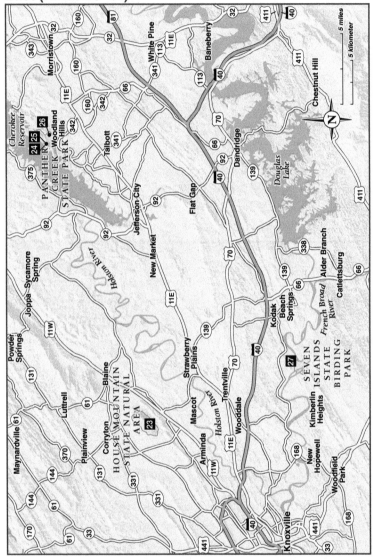

East

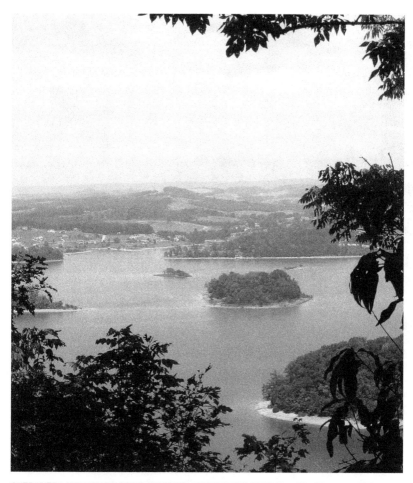

CHEROKEE LAKE VIEWED FROM PANTHER CREEK STATE PARK *(See Hike 25, page 130.)*

23　House Mountain Loop

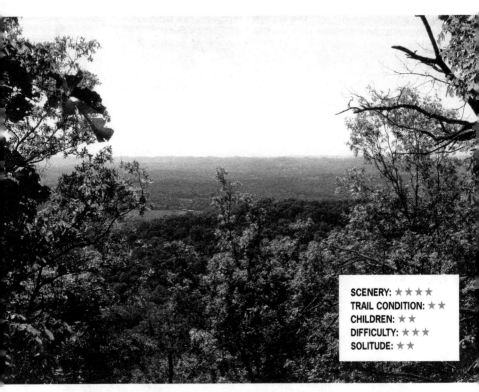

SPECTACULAR VIEWS AWAIT ON MANY HIKES EAST OF KNOXVILLE.

> SCENERY: ★ ★ ★ ★
> TRAIL CONDITION: ★ ★
> CHILDREN: ★ ★
> DIFFICULTY: ★ ★ ★
> SOLITUDE: ★ ★

GPS TRAILHEAD COORDINATES: N36° 06.286' W83° 45.775'

DISTANCE & CONFIGURATION: 2.9-mile loop

HIKING TIME: 1.8 hours

HIGHLIGHTS: Mountain vistas, birding area

ELEVATION: 1,200' at trailhead, 1,950' at West Overlook

ACCESS: No fees, permits, or passes required; open daily sunrise–sunset

MAPS: House Mountain State Natural Area map (see website below), USGS *John Sevier*

FACILITIES: Restrooms and shaded picnic shelter at trailhead

WHEELCHAIR ACCESS: None

COMMENTS: The climb from the trailhead to the crest of House Mountain is short but steep. Be mentally prepared. The best hiking conditions will be found when the trails are dry. Also, as this side of House Mountain faces south, it can be brutally hot on a summer afternoon. If visiting during the warm season, try to start your hike in the morning.

CONTACTS: Knox County Parks and Recreation, 865-215-6600, knoxcounty.org/parks/pdfs/housemtn.pdf

Overview

This loop takes you to a pair of vistas atop House Mountain, the highest point in Knox County, which stands in a 500-acre state natural area and is a steep-sloped, very rocky outlier peak. The geology reveals sheer bluffs, big boulders, rock houses, and, of course, stony overlooks where you can see in all four cardinal directions from various points on the mountain. The views attract hikers as well as birders. Be apprised the hike is steep in areas and part of the mountain contains private property.

Route Details

House Mountain is a great addition to the hiking opportunities in greater Knoxville. Area mountain hiking usually takes place on the Cumberland Plateau or in the Smoky Mountains. House Mountain, a lone physiographic entity, used to be part of Clinch Mountain (which you can see from the East Overlook), but over time Big Flat Creek wore away the land, leaving House Mountain to itself. Now, not only can you see the landmarks of East Tennessee from House Mountain—such as the Smokies, downtown Knoxville, and the Cumberlands—but House Mountain is a landmark itself. And yes, it does have a house shape, which can be seen distinctly on I-40 heading east from Knoxville.

The state-owned parcel is managed by Knox County. A restroom and a shaded picnic pavilion enhance the trailhead. Depart from the trailhead on the Connector Trail; Left Sawmill Loop soon leaves left, but you stay straight. Immediately pass under a power line and reenter hardwoods of red maple, white oak, redbud, and hickory.

Reach a trail junction at 0.1 mile. Stay left, joining the West Overlook Trail. You will climb 700 feet in 0.8 mile. The rocky singletrack path makes its way uphill along Hogskin Branch, which drains the southern reaches of House Mountain. Brush may crowd the narrow path in the growing season.

The climb is moderated by numerous switchbacks; it is the actual slope of the mountain that is so steep. The extreme slope is such that erosive runoff is extra damaging. Parts of this trail system have suffered terrible erosion, so please don't shortcut the switchbacks; fences help prevent hikers from doing so.

By 0.5 mile, you have left Hogskin Branch, angling westerly for the west side of House Mountain. By 0.7 mile you are just below the mountain crest in extremely rocky woods of pine, oak, and sassafras, with an irregular stony cliff line standing above. Come alongside a pair of rock houses at 0.8 mile. The first is

121

House Mountain Loop

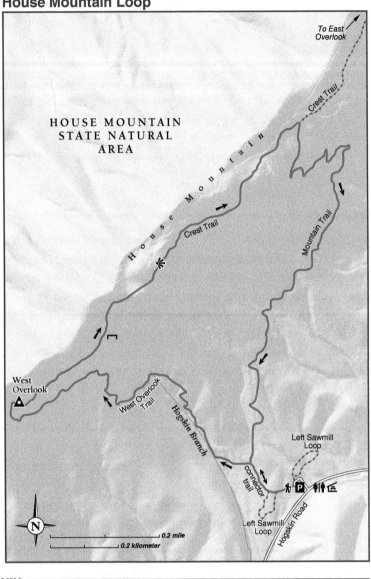

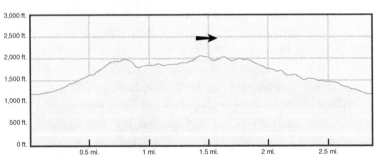

small. Watch for small, gnarled hickory trees clinging to the thin soils between boulders. Views open between the trees to the south. At 0.9 mile the trail curves around the west point of the mountain, angling uphill between boulders to emerge at the West Overlook. Explore a series of multilevel rock protrusions offering vistas primarily to the west, where downtown Knoxville rises.

Beyond the West Overlook, the loop travels east, now on the Crest Trail, through lichen-covered boulders amid cedar, pine, and hickory woods. Obscured views of the Cumberland Plateau open north through the pines. The steep climb is over, and the Crest Trail undulates past a pair of benches at 1.1 miles. The path then picks up an old roadbed and becomes wide and easy as it follows the contours of House Mountain. At 1.3 miles, a short spur trail leads left to a stellar view. Here, hikers are rewarded with clear views of the rolling hills below, Norris Lake in the distance, and Cumberland Mountain rising beyond that. Reach an old roadbed just beyond the overlook, and stay left, wandering under a transmission line. Keep northeast, passing a couple of old roads leading left; one is to private property.

The path descends on a sand, clay, and dirt path to reach a trail junction at 1.7 miles. Here, the Crest Trail continues 0.7 mile to the East Overlook, where you can see Clinch Mountain and beyond; however, the trail runs near private property and you may see ATV riders. Please don't harass them, and respect private property rights. Our loop turns right at the trail junction and descends on the Mountain Trail. The slope shortly becomes insanely steep, and the single-track trail does the best it can to mitigate the slope with switchbacks that navigate wooded rock bluffs.

Views of the Smoky Mountains open to the south. The going is slow, so just take your time and enjoy the views. At 2.1 miles, pass a closed mountain-access trail coming from the lowlands. At 2.3 miles, the trail briefly turns uphill, then bisects the first of several wet-weather streambeds. Watch for big boulders in the woods before completing the loop portion of the hike at 2.8 miles. Backtrack 0.1 mile to the trailhead.

Nearby Attractions

Two short lowland trails emanate from the trailhead: **Left Sawmill Loop** and **Right Sawmill Loop**. Each is about 0.25 mile long, and both travel flats below the mountain, which present wildflowers in early spring.

Directions

From Exit 392 off I-40 east of downtown Knoxville, take US 11W north 10.2 miles to Idumea Road. Turn left on Idumea and follow it 0.6 mile to Hogskin Road. Then turn left on Hogskin Road and follow it 0.7 mile to the trailhead, on your right.

LOOKING DOWN ON KNOX COUNTY AND POINTS BEYOND FROM HOUSE MOUNTAIN

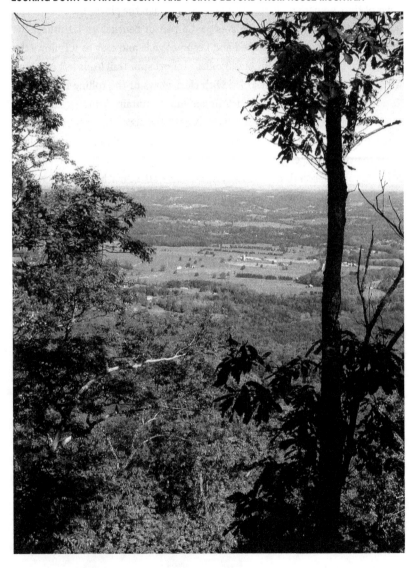

Panther Creek State Park:
Maple Arch Double Loop

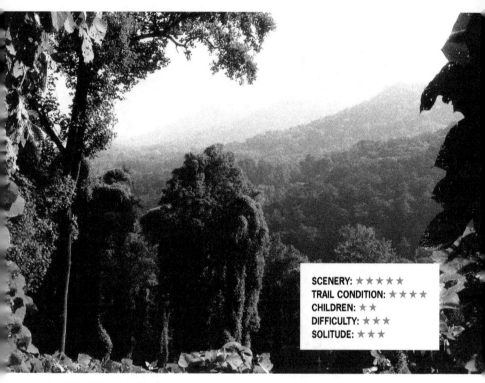

SCENERY: ★ ★ ★ ★ ★
TRAIL CONDITION: ★ ★ ★ ★
CHILDREN: ★ ★
DIFFICULTY: ★ ★ ★
SOLITUDE: ★ ★ ★

KUDZU-COVERED MOUNTAINS

GPS TRAILHEAD COORDINATES: N36° 12.971' W83° 24.338'

DISTANCE & CONFIGURATION: 5.5-mile double loop

HIKING TIME: 2.6 hours

HIGHLIGHTS: Mine vestiges, lake views

ELEVATION: 1,120' at trailhead, 1,410' at high point

ACCESS: No fees, permits, or passes required; park open daily, 8 a.m.–sunset

MAPS: Panther Creek State Park map (see website below), USGS *Talbott*

FACILITIES: The parking area offers restrooms, a covered picnic shelter, and shaded tables.

WHEELCHAIR ACCESS: None

COMMENTS: Avoid this trail on summer weekends, as that is when motorboats and personal watercraft will be tooling noisily all over the place. In winter you will have solitude and also may see waterfowl.

CONTACTS: Panther Creek State Park, 423-587-7046, tnstateparks.com/parks/panther-creek

Panther Creek State Park: Maple Arch Double Loop

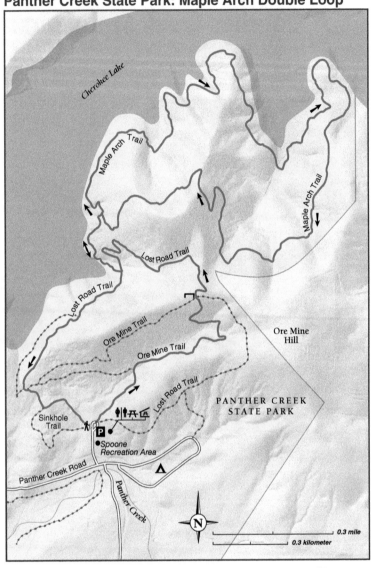

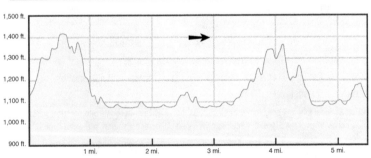

Overview

Make two loops while exploring the hills of Panther Creek State Park, located on the shore of big Cherokee Lake. Follow the Ore Mine Trail up to River Ridge, then drop to the lake's edge. Here, you will trace the shoreline before ascending back into hills. A final stretch takes you past several sinkholes located amidst big wooded boulder fields.

This view-filled hike has many ups and downs, never too long as to be exhausting yet long enough to get your lungs working. During its two-loop trek, the hike passes through numerous environments: lakeshore, boulder fields, cedar thickets, pine woods, cove hardwoods, and even a kudzu stand. The Panther Creek State Park trail system is well signed and maintained.

Route Details

The hike begins with an uphill grade. Pick up Ore Mine Trail at the upper end of the parking area. Pines and cedars rise from the rocky woods. Paw-paws cluster in a draw on trail left, and an impressive boulder field rises to your right. Step over the draw to make a trail junction at 0.2 mile. Stay right with the Ore Mine Trail, continuing up the hollow. It is here you will see shallow pits and gullies from a small-scale, early 1800s manganese-mining operation. Imagine how primitive the extraction techniques were compared to those of today. Trees, vines, and vegetation cover the area, which has recovered well.

Make a sharp switchback at 0.5 mile, trying to surmount River Ridge. The singletrack, hiker-only path tops out on River Ridge at a covered bench and four-way trail junction at 0.7 mile. Take the Lost Road Trail, heading north on a downgrade through maples. It soon turns west toward Cherokee Lake, wandering into boulder-littered hickory, oak, and cedar woods. Avoid the shortcuts other hikers are making as you switchback down the hill. Reach a signed trail junction at 1.2 miles. Turn right here, joining the Maple Arch Trail. Cherokee Lake is now within rock-throwing distance.

The lake is a large TVA impoundment, 29,000 acres large, dammed near Jefferson City and stretching clear up to Rogersville. It is fed by the Holston River and its tributaries. Below the lake dam, the Holston continues into Knoxville, where it meets the French Broad River to form the Tennessee River.

Begin an extended stretch of lakeshore walking. Ahead, at 1.3 miles, spur trails lead left to the water. When the impoundment is below full pool, a gravel beach is exposed here, luring trail users to the lake. At 1.5 miles you will reach the actual loop portion of the Maple Arch Trail. Stay left here, continuing along the shoreline, enjoying lake views as well as vistas of the many islands that rise from the tarn. Curve around a drainage at 1.8 miles. Cedars and scrub pines pock the thin, stony soil. The trail goes off and on old roads abandoned after the Holston River was dammed to create Cherokee Lake.

Lake views persist, with Clinch Mountain as a backdrop. At 2.4 miles, rise from the shoreline as you circle around an embayment. Step over the streambed that creates the embayment at 2.7 miles. Just below the trail, look for the stone remnants of an old primitive bridge crossing the wet-weather stream. Circle around a nearly level peninsula and recovering farm field and homesite. Leave the lakeshore near the park boundary at 3.2 miles. The trail climbs into rocky woods, then passes through a boulder field before entering a moist hollow where the scenery changes yet again to cove hardwoods, such as tulip trees. Vines grow in tangles among the trees. For good measure, the path passes by an invasive stand of kudzu at 4 miles.

Climb via switchbacks away from the weeds over a ridge, then drift west to complete the loop portion of the Maple Arch Trail at 4.6 miles. Be prepared for numerous junctions while working your way back to Spoone Recreation Area. Backtrack 0.2 mile along the lakeshore to rejoin the Lost Road Trail, this time turning right (south), as it scales a hillside well above the water. The trail splits at 5 miles. Stay left with the hiker-only portion of the path through boulders.

Reach a four-way junction at 5.3 miles. Keep straight, still on Lost Road Trail, toward the parking area. You are in an incredible boulder field, surrounded by maple, redbud, hickory, and cedars galore. Reach the Sinkhole Trail at 5.4 miles. You can go right or left on this short loop. A left leads downhill through boulders to a big sink on trail left, at the base of the boulder field. Emerge at the Spoone Recreation Area near the restrooms at 5.5 miles.

Nearby Attractions

The state park has plentiful trails for hikers, bikers, and equestrians; boating; and a campground adjacent to this hike.

Directions

From Knoxville, take US 11E north to Morristown and the intersection of 11E and TN 342 (Panther Creek Road). Turn left on TN 342 West and follow it for

2.4 miles; then turn right into the state park. Keep straight, passing the visitor center. At 0.7 mile, just past the right turn into the campground, turn right into a large parking area at the Spoone shelter. The hike starts at the upper end of the parking area in the auto turnaround.

SHORELINE VIEW OF CHEROKEE LAKE

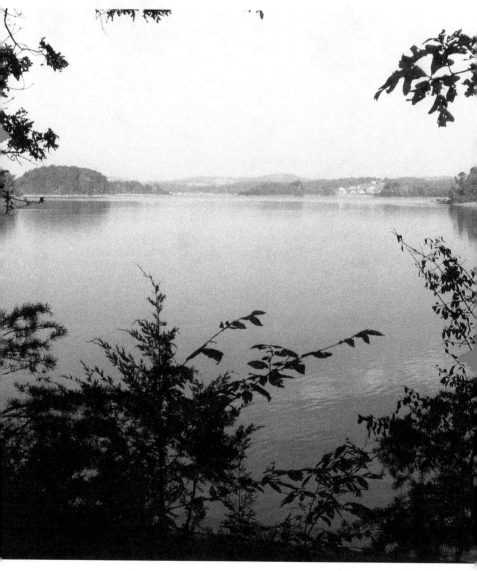

Panther Creek State Park:
Point Lookout Loop

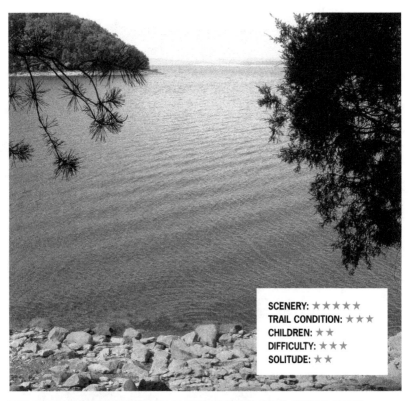

SCENERY: ★ ★ ★ ★ ★
TRAIL CONDITION: ★ ★ ★
CHILDREN: ★ ★
DIFFICULTY: ★ ★ ★
SOLITUDE: ★ ★

VIEW OF CHEROKEE LAKE AFTER THE POSTSUMMER LAKE DRAWDOWN HAS BEGUN

GPS TRAILHEAD COORDINATES: N36° 12.633' W83° 25.387'

DISTANCE & CONFIGURATION: 5.1-mile loop

HIKING TIME: 2.5 hours

HIGHLIGHTS: Multiple lake views from shoreline and hilltops

ELEVATION: 1,290' at trailhead, 1,470' at high point

ACCESS: No fees, permits, or passes required; park open daily, 8 a.m.–sunset

MAPS: Panther Creek State Park map (see website below), USGS *Talbott*

FACILITIES: Restrooms, picnic shelter, picnic area

WHEELCHAIR ACCESS: None

COMMENTS: The state park has miles of additional trails. Bring a meal to enjoy at the trailhead picnic area.

CONTACTS: Panther Creek State Park, 423-587-7046, tnstateparks.com/parks/panther-creek

Overview

This view-laden trek starts with a trip through an amazing boulder garden on a slender but steep peninsula before dropping to Cherokee Lake. Drink in the watery vista before turning up the Panther Creek embayment. Make a side trip to another shoreline with a view. Next, climb a high knob to absorb a first-rate panorama over the lake and beyond to the mountains from aptly named Point Lookout. A final short road walk through an elongated picnic area takes you back to your vehicle. Bring a meal for before or after your hike to enjoy at the trailhead picnic area.

Route Details

Pick up Ridge Crest Trail at the western dead-end turnaround of Smallman Recreation Area. You will have to walk a bit from the parking area to reach the actual trail beginning. Enter a wooded boulder garden, where pale rocks rise from a spare, gnarled forest of cedar, oak, and hickory. Watch for cacti growing in the thin, fast-draining soils. Surmount a knob, then resume a downgrade, meeting the Hunt Knob Trail. Keep straight to the lake and point of the peninsula, reaching a waterside vista at 0.7 mile. A gravel and rock drop-off allows you to access the lake, whether it is at full summer pool or lower winter levels. Stay left on the slender track, keeping the lake to your right, enjoying more aquatic views from the slope of a hill. Turn easterly into the ever-narrowing Panther Creek embayment. At 1.4 miles, the so-called Short Loop leaves left and circles back toward Ridge Crest Trail.

Pass a big sinkhole on the left at 1.5 miles. Traverse some rugged boulder fields between shallow drainages. At 1.7 miles, just before a drainage, look on the right for a rock cavity worn through at the bottom. Technically, this is an arch, but it may only be recognized as such by geologists. Look for willow trees growing in the upper Panther Creek embayment. Ahead, the slope eases. At 2.1 miles, the loop portion of Hunt Knob Trail leaves to the left. Keep straight, passing within earshot of flowing Panther Creek before turning into a grassy meadow and a trail junction at 2.3 miles. Stay left here, crossing the park road you drove in on.

Soon you'll reach yet another trail intersection. Here, Point Lookout Trail begins its loop, heading left or straight. Keep straight, tracing a wide gravel track on a gentle uptick in shady woods. Top out in a gap and trail junction at 2.5 miles. Stay left on Point Lookout Trail, gaining ground to reach a split at

Panther Creek State Park: Point Lookout Loop

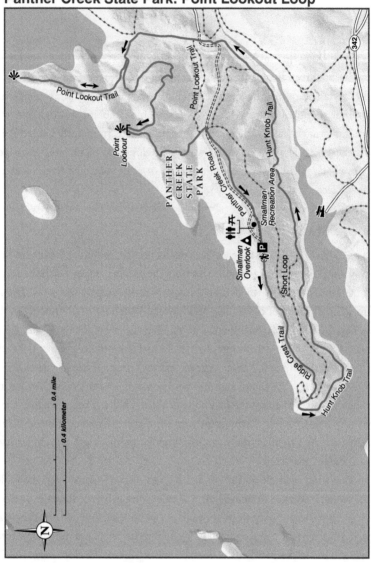

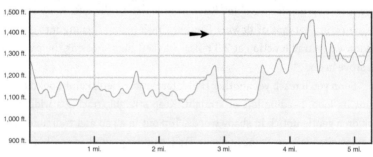

2.7 miles. Here, enjoy your choice of views. Turn right, aiming for an isolated peninsula jutting north into Cherokee Lake. This half-mile spur ends at a point where you can gaze toward islands and beyond to the far lakeshore. This makes a great picnic spot if you want to have lunch on the trail. A gravel beach grown up with persimmon trees is exposed when lake levels are low in winter. Remember this view to contrast it with your next vista, 400 feet higher. Backtrack uphill to the Point Lookout Loop, resuming a climb and breaking through a boulder field at 4 miles. Continue the uptick in maples, reaching Point Lookout at 4.3 miles. Here, a covered bench offers a seat. Soak in panoramas opening to the northwest, of the island-studded impoundment and Clinch Mountain beyond. The vista is easily worth the ascent.

Cruise southwesterly toward the trailhead, meandering downhill to reach a gap and trail junction at 4.7 miles. Here, the other end of Point Lookout Trail comes in from your left. However, this hike keeps straight to shortly emerge on the park road that brought you in. Turn right here, walking west along a grassy roadside strip. The first picnic area loop is just ahead, while the second picnic area loop, with Smallman Overlook, is reached at 5.1 miles, ending the hike.

Nearby Attractions

The state park has plentiful trails for hikers, bikers, and equestrians; boating; and a campground adjacent to this hike.

Directions

From Knoxville, take US 11E north to Morristown and the intersection with TN 342 (Panther Creek Road). Turn left on TN 342 West and follow it 2.4 miles; then turn right into the state park. Keep straight, passing the visitor center. Continue past the campground to reach Smallman Recreation Area after 1.8 miles; then continue past Smallman Overlook to park. *Note:* No parking is allowed in the auto turnaround at the actual trailhead.

26 **Panther Creek State Park:**

Pioneer Loop

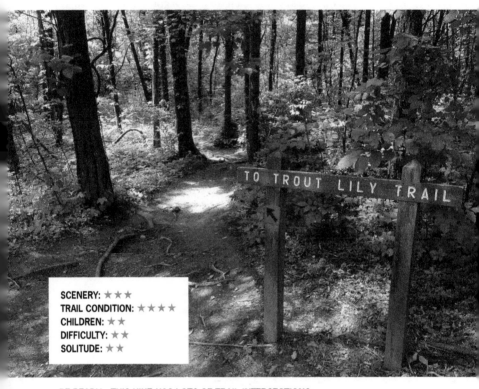

SCENERY: ★ ★ ★
TRAIL CONDITION: ★ ★ ★ ★
CHILDREN: ★ ★
DIFFICULTY: ★ ★
SOLITUDE: ★ ★

BE READY—THIS HIKE HAS LOTS OF TRAIL INTERSECTIONS.

GPS TRAILHEAD COORDINATES: N36° 12.361' W83° 25.126'

DISTANCE & CONFIGURATION: 5.2-mile double loop

HIKING TIME: 2.7 hours

OUTSTANDING FEATURES: Gorgeous forest, lake views

ELEVATION: 1,090' at trailhead, 1,275' at high point

ACCESS: No fees, permits, or passes required; park open daily, 8 a.m.–sunset

MAPS: Panther Creek State Park map (see website below), USGS *Talbott*

FACILITIES: Boat ramp at trailhead; restrooms, picnic shelter, and picnic area at park but not at trailhead

WHEELCHAIR ACCESS: None

COMMENTS: A plethora of trail junctions will keep you studying the trail map—either bring the state park map with you or snap a photo of the map in this guide before you start the hike.

CONTACTS: Panther Creek State Park, 423-587-7046, tnstateparks.com/parks/panther-creek

Overview

This rolling lakeside and hilltop route rolls by the Panther Creek embayment of Cherokee Lake before climbing into a striking hardwood forest and then heading back to the trailhead. Between the wildflowers of spring and the hardwood colors of autumn, the hike presents a new look each season.

Route Details

This view-filled hike has many ups and downs, never too long as to be exhausting yet long enough to get your lungs working. And the scenery meets the standard expected by hikers of Tennessee state parks. Although trails of this hike are ostensibly open to mountain bikers and even another segment is open to equestrians, they are mostly used by hikers. In my wanderings here, I've seen few mountain bikers on the trail, and nary a hoof print.

I do like the challenge and variety of this adventure. The trek meanders along the shore of Cherokee Lake, then comes to a stony segment below partly wooded bluffs that keep you on your toes. And the hills get your lungs going without being so high as to be demoralizing. And upon reaching the Pioneer Trail, savor an opportunity for solitude while walking amid a regal maple-and-oak woodland that comprises as fine a forested stretch as you will experience.

From the boat-ramp parking area, pick up the trail leaving from the top of the loop road, where a sign states TO LILY TRAIL. The singletrack path cruises bottomland rich with cedars, hickories, and pines, with a thick, brushy understory. At 0.1 mile, reach a pair of trail intersections. Stay right at both, beginning a counterclockwise loop of the Trout Lily Trail, named for the yellow wildflower with mottled green leaves resembling the skin of a trout. These diminutive lilies often grow in large colonies in moist hardwood forests, stream valleys, and floodplains in the southeastern United States.

Begin working toward the lakeshore and the Panther Creek embayment of big Cherokee Lake. By 0.3 mile, you're within sight of the shore, winding into and out of little drainages. At 0.7 mile, a land bridge takes you by a steep, seeping bluff. The shoreline becomes more rugged and rocky. Watch your footing. Boardwalks enable other rocky passages. At 0.9 mile, you can peer into Cherokee Lake, 45 square miles in size. The path turns away from the lake and up a draw to reach an intersection at 1.1 miles. Here, head left, climbing, still on the Trout Lily Trail in much less rocky terrain, where you surmount a knob and return nearly to where you just turned left.

Panther Creek State Park: Pioneer Loop

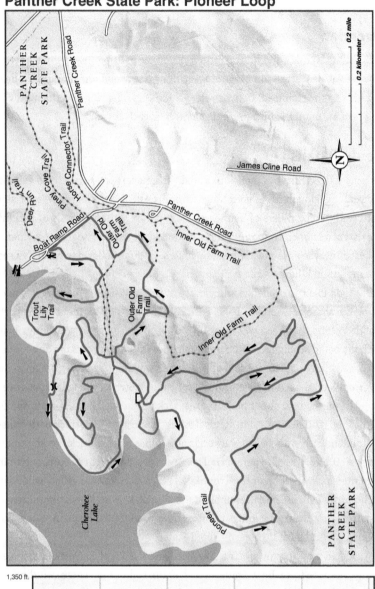

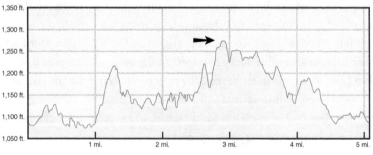

Now, keep southwest in a series of short unnamed connectors to join the Pioneer Trail, a wide former road under cedars, rising to a four-way trail intersection with a shaded bench at 2 miles. Head right on the Pioneer Trail, cruising a slope well above Cherokee Lake. This path is less used. Hike among white oak, maple, and beech. At 2.5 miles, look for signs of an old homesite below the trail. Curve up a hill and enter beautiful forest where hardwoods rise thick overhead, shading a forest floor nearly devoid of ground cover. Look for sinkholes while in this scenic wood deserving of state park status. Reach the ridgetop at 3.2 miles, near another old homesite in a relic clearing. Look for deer in this area. The path then winds near the park boundary a few times while descending to complete the Pioneer Trail at 4.3 miles, back at the four-way intersection.

Now you begin a series of potentially confusing intersections—at this point, break out your map, phone, GPS, set of tarot cards, and rabbit's foot. Head right (east) on the Outer Old Farm Trail to make another intersection at 4.4 miles. Keep straight, still on the Outer Old Farm Trail, descending to thickly wooded bottoms. The land is flatter here, and you come to yet another intersection at 4.6 miles. Go left here, toward the Horse and Bike Trail parking, as the Inner Old Farm Trail loops right. At 4.7 miles, stay left, back on the Outer Old Farm Trail. The brushy, viney woods are dense in these parts, making navigation more difficult. Come to yet another intersection at 4.8 miles. You should see a sign pointing to Boat Ramp Road. Head right here and emerge on Boat Ramp Road at 5 miles, having escaped the clutches of the Outer and Inner Old Farm Trails. Head left, downhill toward the boat ramp, completing the hike at 5.2 miles. Each successive trek on this trail will make it easier to navigate.

Nearby Attractions

The boat ramp at the trailhead offers passage to scenic **Cherokee Lake,** an island-studded impoundment of the Holston River.

Directions

From Knoxville, take US 11E north to Morristown and the intersection with TN 342 (Panther Creek Road). Turn left on TN 342 West and follow it 2.4 miles, passing the right turn into Panther Creek State Park. Keep straight on TN 342 West for 0.5 mile farther, then turn right onto Boat Ramp Road. Follow Boat Ramp Road for 0.4 mile to its dead end at the boat ramp. The hike starts at the upper end of the parking area, just before the loop at the road's end.

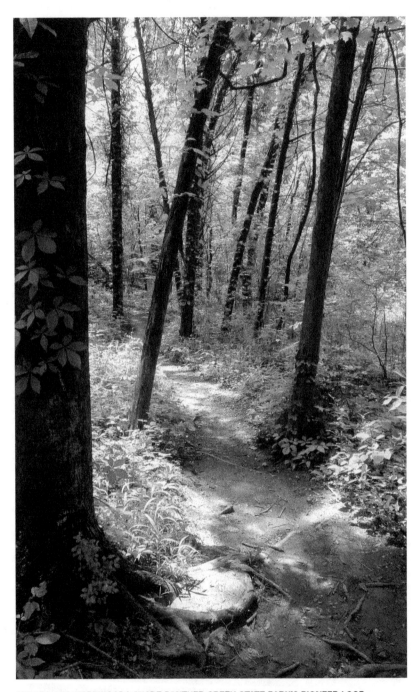

CEDARS AND HARDWOODS SHADE PANTHER CREEK STATE PARK'S PIONEER LOOP.

Seven Islands State Birding Park

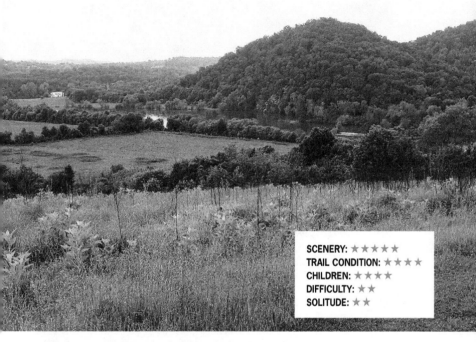

LOOKING DOWN ON THE FRENCH BROAD RIVER AT KELLY BEND

GPS TRAILHEAD COORDINATES: N35° 57.193' W83° 41.224'

DISTANCE & CONFIGURATION: 5.6-mile triple loop, with option to shorten

HIKING TIME: 2.6 hours

OUTSTANDING FEATURES: Birding, views, hiker bridge over French Broad River

ELEVATION: 900' at trailhead, 1,070' at high point

ACCESS: No fees, permits, or passes required; open daily, sunrise–sunset

MAPS: Seven Islands State Birding Park map (see website below), USGS *Boyds Creek*

FACILITIES: Picnic tables, interpretive barn, restrooms near trailhead

WHEELCHAIR ACCESS: Yes, on trail to Seven Islands

COMMENTS: Park offers potential sightings of more than 190 birds. Much of the hike is in the open, so prepare for sun; summer can be hot.

CONTACTS: Seven Islands State Birding Park, 865-407-8335, tnstateparks.com/parks/seven-islands

Seven Islands State Birding Park

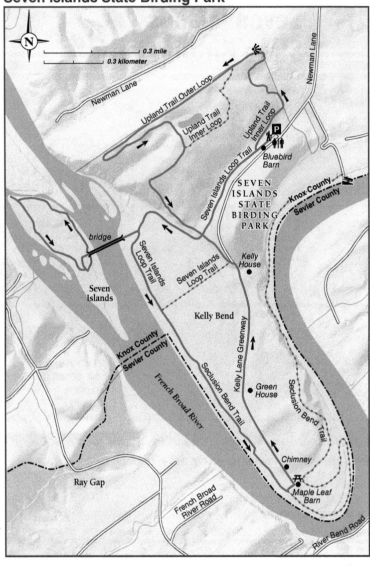

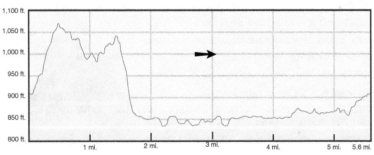

Overview

Enjoy the views, variety, and birding at this wonderful state park located on a bend of the French Broad River. First, climb to a view of the Smokies, then cruise woods and fields before dropping to pick up a track bridging the French Broad River to the Seven Islands. Next, walk the banks of the French Broad before turning up Kelly Lane Greenway, passing a historic house and barns.

Route Details

This first-rate hiking experience presents a variety of sights and scenes—and trails—at this 56th Tennessee state park, established in 2013 and enhanced in 2019 with a hiker bridge over the French Broad River to the Seven Islands, adding one more highlight to the trek. Culled from the historic Kelly Farm (Kellys still live on-site) on appropriately named Kelly Bend, Seven Islands State Birding Park is managed for wildlife while being used as an outdoor education facility, where even average hikers like us can learn a few things about the native flora and fauna of the wildlife preserve. Groups are guided through the park for educational purposes on a regular basis.

You will find the trail system in excellent condition, well marked and maintained. And with the addition of the all-access asphalt path from the trailhead to the Seven Islands in late 2019, a good trail system became great. The bridge provides intimate looks at the French Broad River and enables a loop around the largest of the Seven Islands—the cherry on top of a stellar trail experience.

Start the trek at the Bluebird Barn, an open-air wood structure chock-full of interpretive information. Walk just a few feet, then head right on the Upland Trail Inner Loop on a grassy track that mostly borders woods. Climb past old fencelines, now treelines. The mix of woods and meadow is ideal for wildlife. Bird boxes are common. By 0.5 mile you've done the only climb of the hike and are at a resting bench with a first-rate view south of the crest of the Smokies, highlighted by Mount Le Conte. What a start!

Now, trek along the park boundary between a line of trees and meadows managed for native grasses and wildlife. At 0.6 mile, the Upland Trail Inner Loop splits left, but we stay straight, joining the Upland Trail Outer Loop, still on the highest ridge of the refuge. Curve away from the river, then enter woods, passing a small pond to your left just before coming to another intersection at 1.4 miles, meeting the other end of the Upland Trail Inner Loop. Head right here, back toward the river, enjoying resplendent postcard panoramas of the French Broad and adjacent knobs and bluffs, all framed by the grandiose Smoky Mountains in the distance.

Come to a trail intersection at 1.7 miles. An old road/trail goes right, but you stay left, joining the Seven Islands Loop Trail to reach an intersection at 1.8 miles. Here, hit the asphalt all-access trail leading to Seven Islands. Follow this track through river bottoms of native grasses, coming to the bridge over the French Broad at 2.1 miles. Keep straight, soaking in aquatic vistas while crossing the span. This is a spot worth stopping at for a bit. After reaching the largest of the Seven Islands, head right, making a counterclockwise loop on the wooded isle as the French Broad rushes by. Check out other smaller isles and the far bank. At 2.7 miles, a spur goes to the north point of the island. You are 15 river miles up the French Broad from where it joins the Holston to form the mighty Tennessee River.

Finish the loop and recross the French Broad, once again gazing up and downstream. From here, pick up the Seven Islands Loop Trail, following the riverbank upstream, along a screen of trees, reaching a trail intersection at 3.6 miles. Here, the Seven Islands Loop Trail heads left and away from the river, but we keep straight, joining the Seclusion Bend Trail, following Kelly Bend. The trail was named after what the Kelly family referred to their farm as—Seclusion Bend. Bluffs and bottoms alternate along the far bank. The walking is fine.

At 4.3 miles, take the short spur going left to Kelly Lane Greenway and the Maple Leaf Barn, where shaded picnic tables lie and where I've sat out a thunderstorm. Head up Kelly Lane Greenway, an old paved road with easy walking. Pass a lone chimney, then reach the Green House at 4.7 miles. The home is open to visitors and can be explored.

Kelly Lane Greenway leads you past the Kelly House, still occupied by heirs to this farm; then you reach an intersection at 5.1 miles. Here, drop left onto natural-surface path, rejoining the Seven Islands Loop Trail to emerge at the asphalt all-access trail to the Seven Islands at 5.3 miles. Head right here, climbing through open meadows, and pass the park restrooms before returning to the interpretive Bluebird Barn and the trailhead at 5.6 miles.

Nearby Attractions

The park also has a boat launch that is part of the French Broad River Blueway.

Directions

From Exit 407 off I-40 east of Knoxville, follow Midway Road south 2.6 miles, then turn left on Kodak Road. Follow it 0.4 mile, then turn right onto Kelly Lane. Follow it 0.5 mile to the trailhead at Seven Islands State Birding Park. *Note:* Do not turn left onto the state park boat-ramp road from Kelly Lane; instead, follow Kelly Lane to its end.

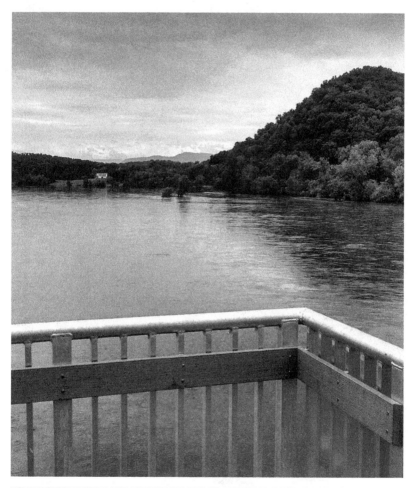

VIEW UPSTREAM FROM THE PEDESTRIAN BRIDGE ACROSS THE FRENCH BROAD RIVER

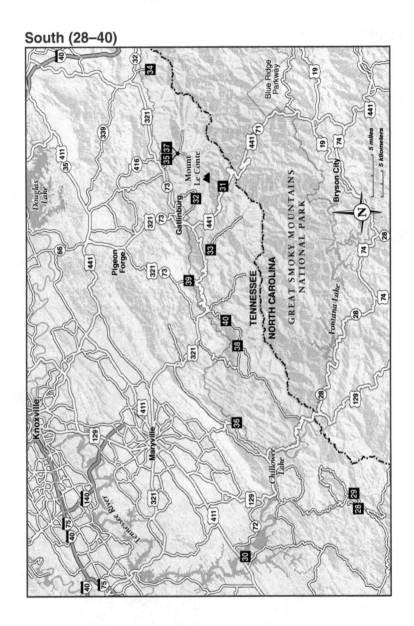

South

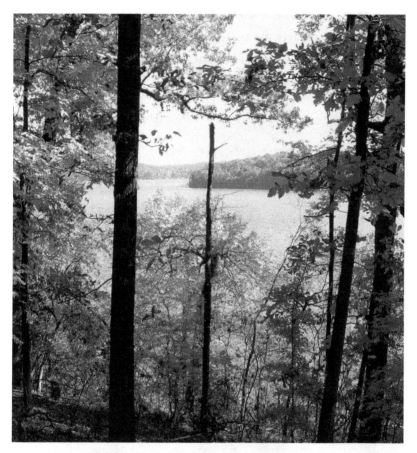

FALL COLOR AT FORT LOUDOUN STATE HISTORIC PARK *(See Hike 30, page 156.)*

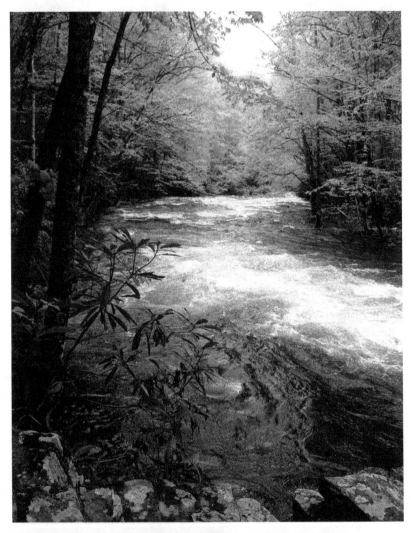

CUCUMBER GAP LOOP IN THE SMOKY MOUNTAINS *(See Hike 33, page 168.)*

28 Cherokee National Forest:
Indian Boundary Lake Loop

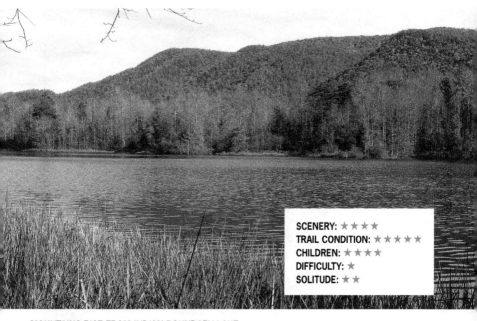

SCENERY: ★ ★ ★ ★
TRAIL CONDITION: ★ ★ ★ ★ ★
CHILDREN: ★ ★ ★ ★
DIFFICULTY: ★
SOLITUDE: ★ ★

MOUNTAINS RISE FROM INDIAN BOUNDARY LAKE.

GPS TRAILHEAD COORDINATES: N35° 23.915' W84° 06.657'

DISTANCE & CONFIGURATION: 3.1-mile loop

HIKING TIME: 1.5 hours

HIGHLIGHTS: Lake and mountain views in an outstanding recreation area

ELEVATION: 1,780' at trailhead, 1,800' at high point

ACCESS: Day-use fee required if not camping; open daily, 8 a.m.–sunset; campground open April–October

MAPS: National Geographic's Trails Illustrated *Tellico & Ocoee Rivers*, USGS *Whiteoak Flats*

FACILITIES: Restrooms and water at picnic area and campground

WHEELCHAIR ACCESS: Yes, all-access trail

CONTACTS: Cherokee National Forest, Tellico Ranger District, 423-397-8455, fs.usda.gov/cherokee

Overview

Make a loop at this scenic Cherokee National Forest impoundment, located in Whiteoak Flats below Flats Mountain. Explore Indian Boundary Recreation

Cherokee National Forest:
Indian Boundary Lake Loop

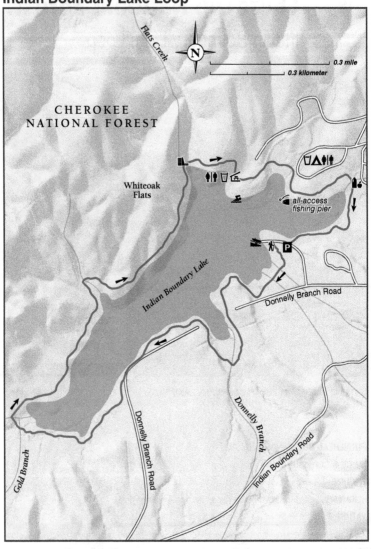

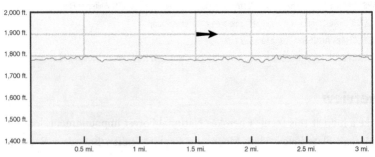

Area via this all-access, nearly level loop trail. Leave the boat ramp and walk past man-made fishing peninsulas, bridging numerous streams shaded in rhododendron. Views open on the lake and on Flats Mountain, which rises on one side of Indian Boundary. You can also enjoy great camping, swimming, and fishing at this mountain retreat.

Route Details

Indian Boundary is the pride of the Cherokee National Forest, and with good reason: the area lies in a flat beside a clear lake and beneath tall mountains. Hikers can enjoy the recreation area on this pleasant and easy loop that's doable by nearly everyone—a great family hike. A coat of pea gravel covers the trail bed, and the scant undulations are graded for wheelchairs. So even when you and the family have polished off a buffet after church, the whole clan could still take on this trail. And from a visual standpoint, you get to enjoy mountain views and scenery without the ruggedness that so often accompanies mountain treks.

Leave the boat ramp, traveling southwesterly, with Indian Boundary Lake to your right. A xeric forest of hickory, pine, sweetgum, and oak shades the level path as it travels through the area known as Whiteoak Flats. And flat it is. Bridge a pair of streamlets at 0.1 mile, then pass through a meadow. Return to the lakeside. You can already look back at the boat ramp and across the lake at the swim beach. Watery views are nearly continuous, albeit sometimes through the trees. Pass the first of several soil fishing peninsulas that extend to the water. Note the nonnative cypress trees planted on these peninsulas.

Bridge Donnelly Branch at 0.5 mile after working around its embayment. Bisect another grassy meadow. These are wildlife clearings maintained by the U.S. Forest Service. These clearings create "edges," where different ecotones overlap, allowing more food for animals. For example, blackberries grow on these edges. Pass an angler's access road at 0.9 mile. At 1 mile, come near gated Donnelly Branch Road, but stay with the pea gravel track and you'll be fine.

Begin circling around the upper lake, bridging Gold Branch and Flats Creek. Watch for evidence of beaver dams here. Turn back northeast. Views open of Flats Mountain rising majestically from the far shoreline. Big white pines shade the path. You are close to the shore and may see paddlers in canoes and kayaks as well as fishermen in johnboats. Circle around an embayment and tributary at 1.8 miles.

At 2.1 miles you are directly across from the boat-ramp trailhead. Bridge the lake dam at 2.2 miles. Come to the swim beach pavilion, with water and restrooms, at 2.4 miles. Begin cruising by the campground, passing coveted lakeside sites. Watch out for social trails leading to camps. Reach the metal all-access fishing pier at 2.6 miles. If you are thirsty, stop at the camp store (open in season) at 2.8 miles. You are in the home stretch. Reach the boat-ramp access road at 3.1 miles, completing the hike.

After seeing Indian Boundary, you may want to camp here. Individual campsites are tastefully integrated into the natural beauty of the land. Amenities include warm showers, electricity at some sites, and flush toilets. Anglers enjoy bank fishing or launching a boat into the clear waters for largemouth bass, trout, and bream. There are purportedly some tackle-busting catfish down deep. You passed the alluring swim beach.

Your entrance road, the Cherohala Skyway, rivals the Blue Ridge Parkway or Newfound Gap Road in the Smokies for scenery. Panoramic overlooks dot the way to Beech Gap and beyond the North Carolina state line. Stop at Hooper Bald. Take a short nature trail to reach this meadow at 5,300 feet in elevation.

Indian Boundary is a popular camping destination. If you want to camp, consider making reservations. A good time to come is May, when spring runs rampant. Fall is also a good choice; the Cherohala Skyway traverses elevations low and high, so leaf viewers are likely to see vibrant colors.

Nearby Attractions

Nearby **Citico Creek Wilderness** (see next hike) offers miles and miles of primitive trails with elevations ranging from 1,100 feet to more than 5,000 feet.

Directions

From Knoxville, take US 129 (Alcoa Highway) south through Maryville and join US 411 south of Maryville, heading to Madisonville. Join TN 68 South to Tellico Plains. From Tellico Plains, pick up TN 165 (Cherohala Skyway) and drive 14 miles to Forest Service Road (FS) 345. Turn left on FS 345 and follow it 1.2 miles into the Indian Boundary Recreation Area. Enter the recreation area, then turn left at a split toward the boat ramp. Turn into the boat-ramp area and park there. The trail leaves left from the boat ramp as you face Indian Boundary Lake.

29 **Cherokee National Forest:**
South Fork Citico Sampler

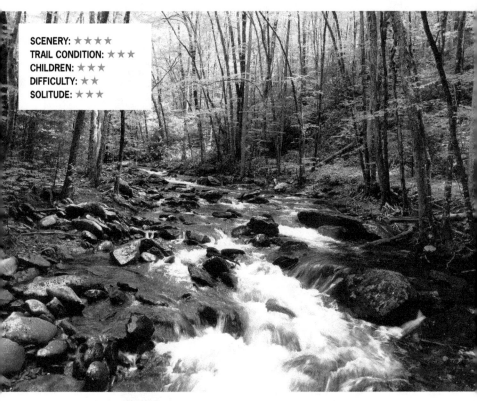

SCENERY: ★ ★ ★ ★
TRAIL CONDITION: ★ ★ ★
CHILDREN: ★ ★ ★
DIFFICULTY: ★ ★
SOLITUDE: ★ ★ ★

SOUTH FORK CITICO CREEK IS A QUINTESSENTIAL MOUNTAIN STREAM.

GPS TRAILHEAD COORDINATES: N35° 24.335' W84° 04.801'

DISTANCE & CONFIGURATION: 3.8-mile out-and-back

HIKING TIME: 2 hours

HIGHLIGHTS: Wilderness stream, swimming, fishing

ELEVATION: 1,720' at trailhead; 2,040' at turnaround point

ACCESS: No fees, permits, or passes required; open year-round, 24-7

MAPS: National Geographic's Trails Illustrated *Tellico & Ocoee Rivers;* USGS *Whiteoak Flats*

FACILITIES: Primitive campground near trailhead

WHEELCHAIR ACCESS: None

CONTACTS: Cherokee National Forest, Tellico Ranger District, 423-397-8455, fs.usda.gov/cherokee

Cherokee National Forest:
South Fork Citico Sampler

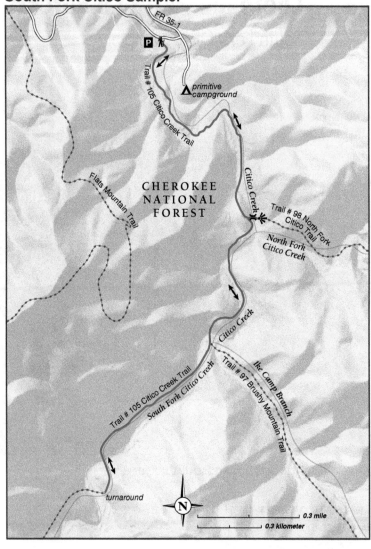

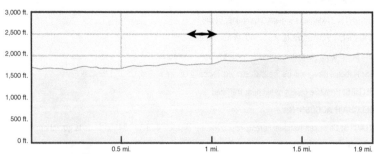

Overview

This hike explores the lowermost part of the gorgeous Citico Creek Wilderness, just south of the Smokies. Follow a trail past the confluence of North and South Fork Citico Creek. Continue up South Fork Citico Creek, with its continuous cascades, rapids, and shoals pouring over rocks and boulders into still, deep pools. The hike wanders up the valley for nearly 2 miles. As no stream fords are required for this part of the trail, you can enjoy it during all seasons—winter with its icy cascades, summer for swimming, spring for wildflowers, and fall for colors.

Route Details

This hike will tempt you to go beyond the mileage recommended in this book—it is that beautiful. South Fork Citico Creek is the centerpiece of the Citico Creek Wilderness. Located just south of Great Smoky Mountains National Park, the area offers scenery like the Smokies minus the crowds. However, the trails are a little rougher, and this lends a more primitive experience overall. That said, you will likely find the experience a good one and want to investigate not only this trail but also other pathways in the 57-mile Citico Creek Wilderness system.

At the trailhead, pass around the vehicle barriers, joining Trail #105. Descend on a doubletrack into a flat. A primitive camping area lies across the creek and is accessed by the concrete ford mentioned in the trailhead directions (page 155). Hikers often start at the primitive campground but end up having to ford Citico Creek to join the official trail.

After 0.25 mile, the path crosses a small rocky tributary. This path slims to a singletrack trail that soon becomes pinched by a steep bluff. Slip down to the water's edge, and look at the creek—rushing rapids fighting their way amidst mossy gray boulders, water striders standing on the surface of still eddies, fallen trees being ceaselessly pushed by the current, and bubbles from white froth oxygenating the water for wily trout. Vegetation grows to the shoreline, forming a natural green tunnel for Citico Creek. The sun penetrates where the stream is at its widest and when the fallen leaves allow weak winter rays to shine through the translucent water—a classic Southern Appalachian mountain stream within a federally designated wilderness.

While hiking, watch for white quartz rocks brightening the woods. Open into a flat at 0.4 mile. Trees are now growing up in this once brushy area. You may see structure foundations of what was purportedly an orchard. At 0.5 mile, a wooden sign welcomes you into the wilderness. A user-created trail comes in

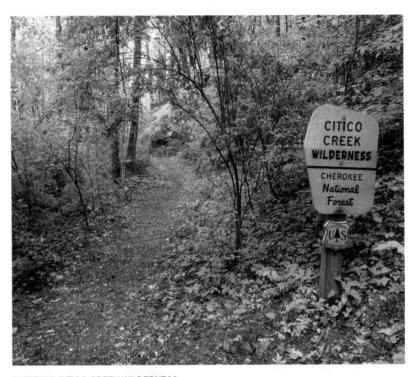

ENTERING CITICO CREEK WILDERNESS

from the primitive campground across the creek. You are back along the stream. Sweetgum, red maple, Fraser magnolia, and sycamore shade the track. White pine, doghobble, and rhododendron add an evergreen touch to the biodiversity.

The ultraclear water repeatedly lures you toward Citico Creek. At 0.7 mile, big, open rock slabs beside some rapids provide the perfect opportunity to get close to the stream. Ahead, turn away from the creek. Even when you can't see the stream, it is always within earshot. Join an old railroad grade. Unbelievably, this area was once connected to Maryville by rail. A logging company built the system to extract timber from the Citico Creek watershed. Just ahead, you'll see a concrete building on your right. It is all that remains of the logging community of Jeffrey. Operations ceased in the 1920s when a huge fire burned up the infrastructure and woodlands. A few years later the area was purchased by the U.S. Forest Service, and over the decades it has healed into a land of spring wildflowers, summertime trout fishing, and a fall kaleidoscope of color.

At 0.8 mile, come to a trail junction. Here, the North Fork Citico Trail, Trail #98, leaves left. Go ahead and take the trail and reach a bridge over Citico Creek. This offers an overhead vista of the mountain rill. North Fork and South Fork merge just below the bridge. Return to the South Fork Trail, Trail #105, and continue upstream, now tracing South Fork Citico Creek.

The tread has narrowed and you follow the old railroad bed. The unbroken beauty continues in pools and shoals. At 1.2 miles, you can see Ike Camp Branch splashing its way to meet Citico Creek. At 1.3 miles, Brushy Mountain Trail, Trail #97, heads left but requires a ford of South Fork. Continue upstream. At 1.9 miles, the trail leads directly to an old ford of Citico Creek. This is a good place to turn around. However, a slender footpath leaves right, climbs a hill, and descends back to the creek, getting around two old fords and rejoining the old railroad grade after 0.5 mile before reaching the first mandatory ford of Citico Creek. On your return trip, find a good riverside rock and enjoy this watery jewel of East Tennessee.

Nearby Attractions

Nearby **Citico Wilderness** offers many miles of primitive trails and first-rate backpacking with elevations ranging from 1,100 feet to more than 5,000 feet.

Directions

From Knoxville, take US 129 (Alcoa Highway) south through Maryville and join US 411 south of Maryville, heading toward Madisonville. Bridge the impounded Tellico River, coming to Vonore. Look for the intersection with TN 360 at a traffic light. Turn left on TN 360 South, and drive 12.9 miles to County Road 504 (Chestnut Valley Road, also known as Buck Highway). A sign to Citico Creek will mark your left turn. After the left turn, drive 5.1 miles to Forest Service Road (FS) 35-1/Citico Creek Road. Turn right on FS 35-1, passing Doublecamp camping area at 6.4 miles. Keep straight here, crossing a bridge. At 8 miles, FS 35-1 makes a sharp right turn—a road splits left to a concrete ford over Citico Creek and Citico Creek Camping Area #14, but do not take that road; instead, continue uphill 0.1 mile farther to the South Fork Citico Trail (Trail #105) trailhead. It is on your left, with a pair of big rock vehicle barriers. There is parking for one or two cars near the gate or beside the road. If this area is somehow full, you can park at the primitive campground across the concrete ford.

30

Fort Loudoun
State Historic Park

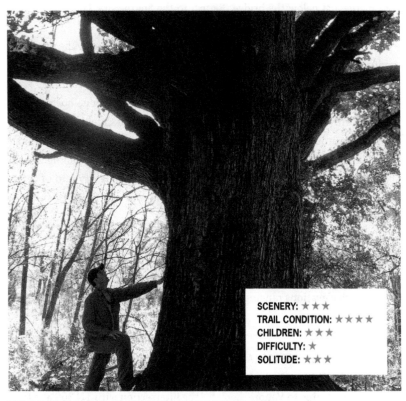

SCENERY: ★ ★ ★
TRAIL CONDITION: ★ ★ ★ ★
CHILDREN: ★ ★ ★
DIFFICULTY: ★
SOLITUDE: ★ ★ ★

THIS OAK WAS AROUND BEFORE TENNESSEE BECAME A STATE.

GPS TRAILHEAD COORDINATES: N35° 35.651' W84° 12.510'

DISTANCE & CONFIGURATION: 3.4-mile loop

HIKING TIME: 2 hours

HIGHLIGHTS: Lake views, mountain views, diverse habitats

ELEVATION: 860' at trailhead to 950' at high point

ACCESS: No fees, permits, or passes required; park open daily, 8 a.m.–sunset

MAPS: Fort Loudoun State Historic Park map (see website below), USGS *Vonore*

FACILITIES: Picnic area, water, restrooms, museum near trailhead

WHEELCHAIR ACCESS: None

CONTACTS: Fort Loudoun State Historic Park, 423-420-2331, tnstateparks.com/parks/fort-loudoun

Overview

Make a loop on a water-encircled peninsula at this site of an 18th-century English fort. Leave an attractive picnic area, then travel hilly woods overlooking Tellico Lake. The hike then winds through open meadows before returning waterside. A hill climb leads to rewarding overlooks of the Southern Appalachians. From there, drop to a homesite and massive white oak tree that has to be seen to be believed. Finally, return to the picnic area, where you can incorporate a visit to the park museum/fort into your experience.

Route Details

Pick up the Ridgetop Trail at the kiosk in the picnic area. Travel south through pine, hickory, oak, and cedar woods on a slope. As you are on a peninsula, Tellico Lake is never far. Here, it is off to your left (east) through the trees. On a clear day you can easily see the crest of the Appalachians to the east. The natural-surface singletrack path undulates across drainages leading toward the lake.

Bridge ravines at 0.2 mile and 0.3 mile. At 0.5 mile come to a trail junction. Here, Ridgetop Trail heads right, making a shorter circuit. You stay left, now picking up Meadow Loop Trail. Continue traveling through woods, with a meadow within sight to your right. At 0.8 mile, you will come to another intersection. Here, stay left with Lost Shoe Loop Trail, which leads downhill toward the shoreline. Come directly along the water. The TN 360 bridge comes into view. Climb away from the water, then enter a dense coppice of Virginia pines.

Return to meet Meadow Loop Trail at 1.2 miles, still in pines. Interestingly, the trail dips into a wooded sinkhole. Pass above another sinkhole, enjoying a top-down view. At 1.6 miles, the trail opens into a meadow. Rolling hills are covered with tall, wavy grasses and sporadic trees. The path is easy to follow, as it is mown through the meadow. Look back to the east as you travel through the meadow for views of the state-line ridge and glimpses of Tellico Lake.

Cross the main park road at 1.9 miles. Reenter woods, heavy with sweet-gum trees. Come along the shoreline again, this time on the western side of the peninsula. You're so close to the water that one false step will wet your shoes. Make a northbound track. At 2.4 miles, the path curves abruptly right past an embayment. Begin climbing to the high point of the peninsula, reaching a trail junction at 2.8 miles. Here, rejoin the Ridgetop Trail, which really does travel the ridge top here. Wander through a mix of field and trees on an old farm road.

Fort Loudoun State Historic Park

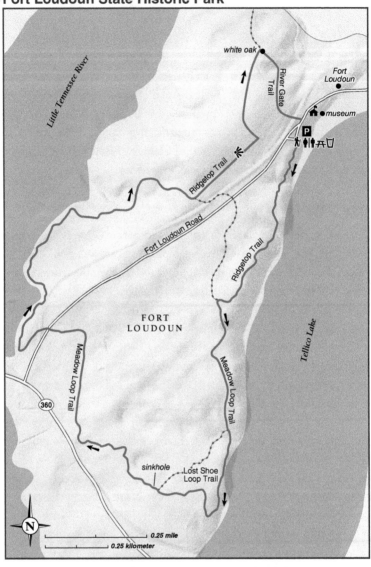

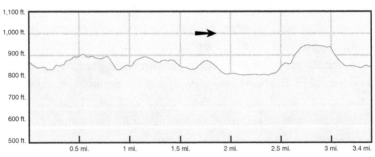

Sweeping views of the Smokies and the Unicoi Mountains south of the Smokies open up above the fields. What a sight!

At 3 miles, the path reenters woods. Dip to reach a trail junction at an old homesite at 3.2 miles. You can't miss what has to be one of the largest white oak trees in the state. The enormous trunk splits into numerous limbs. Leave right from here, joining River Gate Trail on a crumbly asphalt road rendered useless by the flooding of Tellico Lake. This stretch leads you back to the trailhead.

The English built Fort Loudoun here to counter French influence and build relations with the nearby Cherokee during Colonial times. Finished in 1756, the fort saw no military action. However, relations between the British and Cherokee turned out badly. The natives laid siege to the fort from March until August of 1760. The British surrendered and left the fort but were attacked and either killed or captured and enslaved. Eventually, many of the survivors were ransomed and returned to their families. The fort was all but forgotten until the early 1900s, when a marker commemorated the site. In 1933, the land was bought by the state and eventually became the preserve we see today. Visit the park museum for a more in-depth Fort Loudoun learning experience.

Nearby Attractions

While you are here, consider also visiting the **Sequoyah Birthplace Museum**, which is just a short distance down TN 360 on your right. Sequoyah, a Cherokee, invented the Cherokee alphabet and developed the written word for his people. For more information, visit sequoyahmuseum.com.

Directions

From Knoxville, take US 129 (Alcoa Highway) south through Maryville and join US 411 south of Maryville, heading toward Madisonville. After about 15.5 miles, bridge the impounded Tellico River, coming to Vonore. About 1.5 miles farther, look for the intersection with TN 360 at a traffic light. Turn left on TN 360 South and drive 1 mile to Fort Loudoun State Historic Park, on your left. Turn into the park and follow the main park road 1 mile to a picnic area, on your right. Park here. The hike starts at a trailhead kiosk.

31

Smoky Mountains:
Alum Cave Bluffs

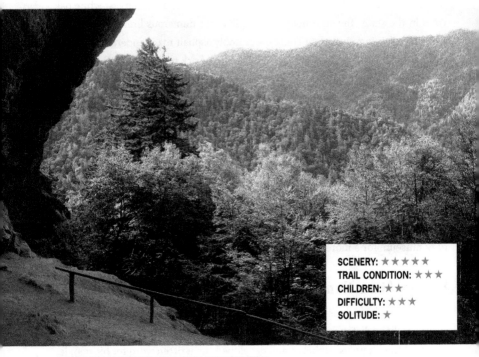

SCENERY: ★ ★ ★ ★ ★
TRAIL CONDITION: ★ ★ ★
CHILDREN: ★ ★
DIFFICULTY: ★ ★ ★
SOLITUDE: ★

ALUM CAVE BLUFFS TRAIL IS BUSY BUT BEAUTIFUL.

GPS TRAILHEAD COORDINATES: N35° 37.690' W83° 27.020'

DISTANCE & CONFIGURATION: 4.6-mile out-and-back

HIKING TIME: 2.6 hours

HIGHLIGHTS: Old-growth trees, great views, natural arch, rock bluff with views

ELEVATION: 3,890' at trailhead, 5,000' at turnaround point

ACCESS: No fees, permits, or passes required; open year-round, 24/7

MAPS: nps.gov/grsm/planyourvisit/maps.htm, USGS *Mount Le Conte*

FACILITIES: None

WHEELCHAIR ACCESS: None

COMMENTS: Try to plan your hike during off times to avoid crowds. I suggest getting there at sunrise, during times of possible rain, or on winter weekdays. Avoid summer or holiday weekends, as Smokies visitors from afar clog this deserving highlight reel of a hike. It also gets use from folks hiking up and down on overnight trips to Mount Le Conte Lodge.

CONTACTS: Great Smoky Mountains National Park, 865-436-1200, nps.gov/grsm

Overview

Some hikes are busy for a reason, and this one has several, including highlights ranging from spectacular views to old-growth forests to a natural arch—rare for the Smokies—and finally to an overhanging bluff with views of its own. If you time your hike right, you can enjoy these highlights on a less crowded trek.

Route Details

The steep slopes of Mount Le Conte contain some of the most beautiful scenery in the Smokies. This hike travels an ancient forest along Alum Cave Creek before turning up Styx Branch, where Arch Rock awaits. This geological feature is different from the classic arches you may have seen on the Cumberland Plateau; it is more of a circular maw, with stone steps leading through it. The hike then opens onto a heath bald where a rock promontory lives up to its name: Inspiration Point. Finally, you climb a rock slope to reach Alum Cave Bluffs, a huge rock overhang with views of its own.

Spur trails from the two large parking areas converge at the bridge over Walker Camp Prong. Old-growth forest of yellow birch and spruce rises above the hiker-only trail as it slices through a rhododendron sea. Bridge Alum Cave Creek on a log. Some of the preserved hemlocks can be seen close to the trailhead, and you will also see red spruce, another evergreen. Watch for a massive red spruce to the left of the trail at 0.4 mile. This is a good spot to look around and take inventory of the grove.

Authentic old-growth woodland is not an agglomeration of ancient trees. On the contrary, even aged trees are a result of disturbance. An old-growth forest will have many big trees, along with younger trees that grow when they get the chance. A growth opportunity is created when a big tree falls, allowing more light in. Young trees sprout in this light gap, and other already somewhat-grown trees thrive in the additional sun. Other times, in the dim of the dark forest, trees may gain a foothold on nurse logs. Nurse logs are fallen and decaying trees that allow a seedling to take root; the young trees are then fed with the energy contained within the decaying log. Later, the new trees grow and spread roots around the fallen log. Over time, the nurse log returns entirely to the soil, and the newly grown tree looks as if it grew up with legs.

The heavily traveled trail is quite rooty, so watch your footing, as well as the stately giants above and the crystalline stream beside you, with its beige, gray, and tan rocks. Cross Alum Cave Creek on another log at mile 1. The trail swerves left

Smoky Mountains: Alum Cave Bluffs

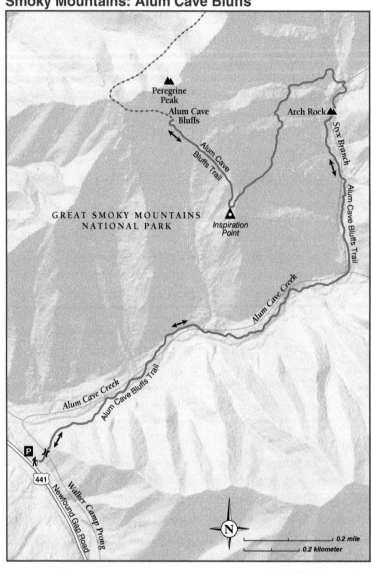

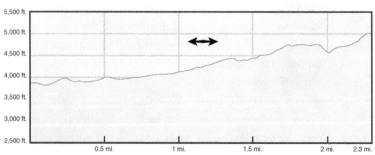

and begins to follow Styx Branch, which it bridges at 1.3 miles. Watch for a gigantic buckeye tree just after this crossing that brings you over to the left (west) bank.

Next come to one of nature's more erosive projects, Arch Rock, at 1.4 miles, just after another log crossing of Styx Branch. At first, it seems that the path dead-ends. However, a set of stone stairs leads the way through the tunnel-like arch. Continue ascending, stepping over Styx Branch a final time at 1.5 miles. Open onto an area covered with small, low bushes, known as a heath bald. Rock outcrops are mixed among the low-slung Catawba rhododendron, sand myrtle, and mountain laurel, along with a few wind-sculpted trees. Interestingly, sand myrtle grows only along the Southeastern coastline and the Southern Appalachians but isn't found in the hundreds of miles between the distinctly different ecosystems.

Views open from Inspiration Point at 2 miles, including the Chimneys and Sugarland Mountain across the gulf; the rockslides of Anakeesta Ridge; and slides nearer to the west, where unstable soils have simply sloughed off the mountainside, usually following heavy rain events. Give yourself ample time to relax in this superlative setting.

Leave the bald, cruising the rock face of Peregrine Peak, a stony knob of Mount Le Conte. Because the mostly open rock trail can get quite icy in winter, the park service has strung wire hand railings along the declivitous slope. Arrive at Alum Cave Bluffs, residing at the 5,000-foot elevation, at 2.3 miles. The rock overhang with a dusty floor really isn't a cave. During the Civil War, soldiers led by Thomas Walker and his band of Confederate Cherokees mined the bluff for saltpeter to make gunpowder for the South. You can usually smell the sulfur in the air at the bluff. In winter, large icicles form at the top of the overhang and crash down when the air warms. Nature is constantly at work on the Alum Cave Bluffs Trail.

Nearby Attractions

The **Sugarlands Visitor Center** offers interpretive information, historic displays, restrooms, and water.

Directions

From the junction of US 321 and US 441/Parkway in Gatlinburg (signed traffic light #3), head south on US 441 for 2.7 miles into the park. With the Sugarlands Visitor Center on your right, keep south on US 441/Newfound Gap Road for 8.9 miles. The Alum Cave Bluffs parking area will be on your left.

32 # Smoky Mountains:
Baskins Creek Loop

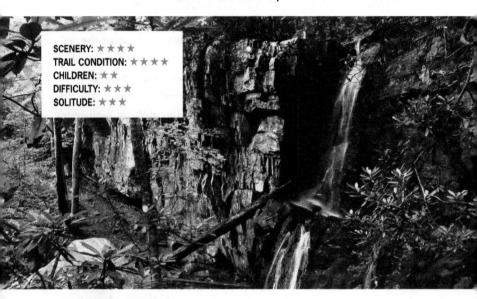

SCENERY: ★ ★ ★ ★
TRAIL CONDITION: ★ ★ ★ ★
CHILDREN: ★ ★
DIFFICULTY: ★ ★ ★
SOLITUDE: ★ ★ ★

BASKINS CREEK FALLS

GPS TRAILHEAD COORDINATES: N35° 40.650' W83° 28.712'

DISTANCE & CONFIGURATION: 6.4-mile loop

HIKING TIME: 3.7 hours

HIGHLIGHTS: Waterfall, views, homesites

ELEVATION: 3,278' at high point, 2,085' at low point

ACCESS: No fees, permits, or passes required; open year-round, 24/7

MAPS: nps.gov/grsm/planyourvisit/maps.htm, USGS *Mount Le Conte*

FACILITIES: None

WHEELCHAIR ACCESS: None

COMMENTS: No pets allowed in park

CONTACTS: Great Smoky Mountains National Park, 865-436-1200, nps.gov/grsm

Overview

This loop, very near Gatlinburg, travels surprisingly hilly terrain and winds amid multiple ecotones to reach Baskins Falls and some pioneer history. The route then meets Roaring Fork Motor Nature Trail. Hikers walk the motor trail a short way to meet Trillium Gap Trail, which returns them to the trailhead.

Route Details

Baskins Creek, home to Smoky Mountains pioneers, doesn't seem a likely settler locale; its numerous hills and tight but small valleys challenged those who
wished to live here in the shadow of Mount Le Conte. Now you can get a good
workout while seeing a little history, plus Baskins Creek Falls. That cascade is
overshadowed by two better-known cataracts, Rainbow Falls and Grotto Falls,
both of which are accessed from this general area. Waterfall enthusiasts could
bag all three in a day. Baskins Creek Falls is by far the least visited of them all.

Finding Baskins Creek Trail can be a challenge. It is best accessed where
it crosses Roaring Fork Motor Nature Trail 0.2 mile beyond that road's beginning, where you should park. Leave left from the motor trail. The hillier-than-
you-think path meanders innocently through second-growth woodland before
turning uphill onto an unnamed pine, oak, and mountain laurel ridge spurring
off Piney Mountain, a shoulder of Mount Le Conte. Views of Cove Mountain
open to the west. Cruise along this eye-catching ridgeline before steeply dropping to meet Falls Branch, a tributary of Baskins Creek. Step over the stream at
1 mile, soon passing a rock overhang on trail right. Overhangs such as this are
uncommon in the Smokies, as opposed to the Cumberland Plateau, west of the
Knoxville, where rock shelters and overhangs are ubiquitous.

Just as the hollow of Falls Branch becomes suffocatingly tight, it widens
and reveals a sea of rhododendron below, where Falls Branch crashes downstream. Though the falls is obscured by the rhododendron, its watery sounds fill
the hollow. The path slips across a small flat to meet a spur trail leading left.
This path travels 0.25 mile uphill to Baskins Cemetery, a small pioneer cemetery.
Baskins Creek Trail continues downstream to meet another spur at 1.3 miles.
This is the path to Baskins Falls. Trace the 0.25-mile spur trail past a pioneer
homesite and down a muddy track. The flat where the homesite stands closes,
and the trail drops steeply to Baskins Falls, which spills over a wide rock face in
two stages. You'll likely be able to enjoy this cataract by yourself, while throngs
crowd Rainbow Falls and Grotto Falls. Interestingly, pioneers purportedly used
Baskins Falls as a natural shower.

Baskins Creek Trail curves over a ridge, then drops to meet Baskins Creek.
Step over the stream and meet an old wagon road that goes in both directions
along Baskins Creek. Follow the track up Baskins Creek, in another tight hollow
made tighter by rhododendron tunneling over the trail. The hollow opens to a
final homesite, the highest on Baskins Creek, before turning up a dry drainage.

Smoky Mountains: Baskins Creek Loop

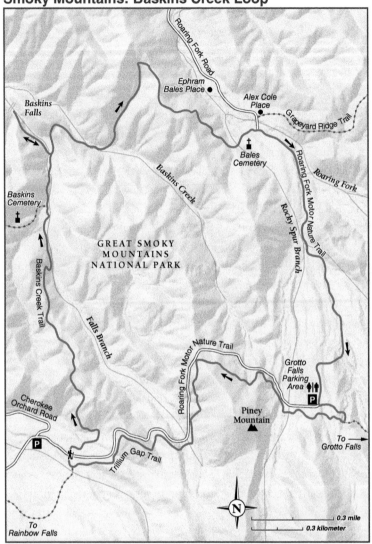

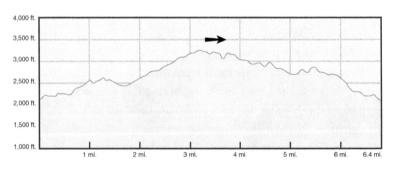

The subsequent 500-foot climb to the ridge dividing Baskins Creek from Rocky Spur Branch is steep. The trail levels out a bit on the ridgeline, where chestnut oaks thrive, to bisect Rocky Spur Branch. Bales Cemetery is just beyond Rocky Spur Branch on your right, enclosed in a fence. Most of the markers are simple unmarked vertical rock slabs. Meet Roaring Fork Motor Nature Trail at 2.7 miles. The Alex Cole homestead is just down the road and across Roaring Fork.

Now turn right, heading up Roaring Fork Motor Nature Trail, watching for cars. Also watch for showy orchis and foamflower in spring. Bridge Rocky Spur Branch at 3.2 miles, then come to the well-used connector path leading to Trillium Gap Trail at 3.9 miles. Turn left and soon reach the Trillium Gap Trail. If you want to extend your loop, go left to Grotto Falls, 1.1 miles distant. Our loop veers right on Trillium Gap Trail. This lesser-used, nearly level path follows an old mountain roadbed, crossing small creeks coming off the side of Mount Le Conte. Doghobble, ferns, and rhododendron border the trail as it passes above the Grotto Falls parking area, which has a restroom. Quartz outcrops brighten the woods. Watch for occasional big trees. The path begins a downgrade before it reaches a trail junction near an incredibly gnarled oak tree. It is but a few feet to the right to reach Roaring Fork Motor Nature Trail and the end of your loop at 6.4 miles.

Nearby Attractions

Gatlinburg is one of East Tennessee's biggest tourist attractions and offers everything from music shows to off-the-wall museums.

Directions

From the junction of US 321 and US 441/Parkway in Gatlinburg (signed traffic light #3), head south and west 0.6 mile on US 441, and turn left on Historic Nature Trail at traffic light #8 for Airport Road. Follow Historic Nature Trail 0.6 mile, and at the intersection keep straight on Cherokee Orchard Road to enter the park. In 1.9 miles, bear right at the fork, and in another 0.9 mile, reach another fork—here, Cherokee Orchard Road keeps straight, while Roaring Fork Motor Nature Trail heads right. Park at this intersection. Walk up Roaring Fork Motor Nature Trail for 0.2 mile to reach the Baskins Creek Trail, on your left. (There is room for one or two cars at the trailhead.) In winter, Roaring Fork Motor Nature Trail will be gated, but you can simply walk around the gate to access the trail.

33 Smoky Mountains:
Cucumber Gap Loop

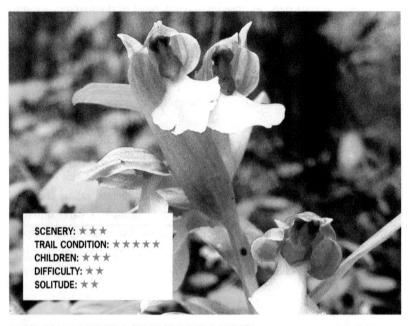

SCENERY: ★ ★ ★
TRAIL CONDITION: ★ ★ ★ ★ ★
CHILDREN: ★ ★ ★
DIFFICULTY: ★ ★
SOLITUDE: ★ ★

SHOWY ORCHIS BRIGHTENS SPRINGTIME IN THE SMOKIES.

GPS TRAILHEAD COORDINATES: N35° 39.218' W83° 34.778'

DISTANCE & CONFIGURATION: 5.6-mile loop

HIKING TIME: 3 hours

HIGHLIGHTS: River views, waterfall, national park–caliber scenery

ELEVATION: 2,200' at trailhead, 2,900' at high point

ACCESS: No fees, permits, or passes required; open year-round, 24/7

MAPS: nps.gov/grsm/planyourvisit/maps.htm, USGS *Gatlinburg*

FACILITIES: Restrooms and water at nearby Elkmont Campground

WHEELCHAIR ACCESS: None

COMMENTS: No pets allowed in national park

CONTACTS: Great Smoky Mountains National Park, 865-436-1200, nps.gov/grsm

Overview

This is an ideal hike for those who want more of a woodland stroll than a lung-busting alpine ascent. Leave the Elkmont area of the park and cruise up the ultra-attractive Little River Valley, where the watercourse tumbles over huge boulders, forming large clear pools that invite a dip in the cool mountain stream. Pass a tributary making a waterfall just as it reaches the Little River. Leave the Little River on an old railroad grade that gently climbs to a gap, then descend to Jakes Creek Valley and return to Elkmont.

Route Details

The Little River drains the highest point in the Smokies, Clingmans Dome, then gathers tributaries, flowing north and west through the park before emerging near the community of Townsend. From there it continues northwest to meet the Tennessee River near Maryville. You'll begin on a path that was part of the Little River Road until a mid-1990s flood washed out this upper section. The park service decided to move the trailhead back rather than repair the road.

Pass through the former Elkmont summer home community, known as the Appalachian Club, on a crumbling asphalt path. Vestiges of the stone entrance gates and summer cottages survive. After 0.25 mile, you leave the old summer cottage community on a wide gravel track shaded by tulip trees, sycamore, black birch, yellow birch, and scads of doghobble and rhododendron mixed with mossy boulders. The sparkling Little River lies to the left, always trying to lure you to its banks with attractive shoals, crystalline pools, small islands, and big rocks ideal for sunning or feeling the cool breeze flow down the valley. At 0.4 mile, Bearwallow Branch comes in on your right.

At 1 mile, the path narrows after you pass the old parking area. A bluff pinches the trail to the river in places. In other spots the Little River is only audible, not visible. Burnt Mountain rises to your right, and this hike leads completely around the wooded peak. At 2 miles, Huskey Branch flows under a bridge into the Little River and a large pool below. Here, Huskey Branch tumbles as a multitiered cascade above and below the trail as it slices through jagged rock. Look into the pool below for swimming trout. Brook trout, technically a char, are the only native trout in the Smokies. However, brown trout and rainbow trout have been introduced into the park, and these are the ones you are most likely to see in the lower Little River.

Keep walking for a bit, coming to an intersection with the Cucumber Gap Trail at 2.4 miles. Turn right onto the Cucumber Gap Trail. This path may have more vines among the trees than any other in the park. Ascend an old railroad grade, rock-hopping Huskey Branch at mile 2.8. Muscadine vines are prominent in the trailside forest. Muscadines, small native grapes, ripen in early fall and

Smoky Mountains: Cucumber Gap Loop

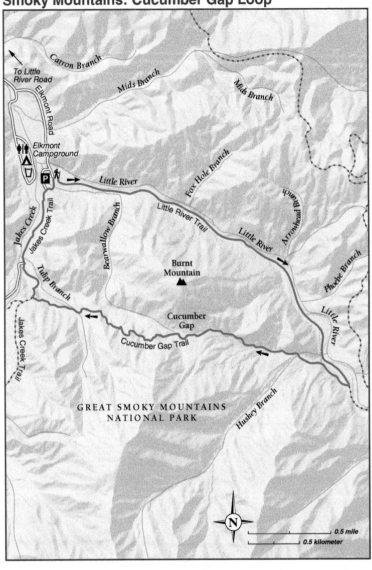

are favored by all sorts of wildlife in the Smokies. The thick-skinned fruit grows throughout the Southeast, and early settlers used it to make wine; today's winemakers purposely cultivate the varietal. The fruit is also touted as a modern-day antioxidant-rich health food.

The path keeps rising along a small feeder stream of Huskey Branch, crossing it at 3.2 miles. Occasional views open through the trees to the right. The path passes just above Cucumber Gap at 3.5 miles; you are just below 3,000 feet. The gap was named for the cucumber tree, which is part of the magnolia family. Its green fruit resembles a mini cucumber and will be seen trailside in September. The tree appears throughout the mid-Appalachians, with West Virginia in the heart of its range. Outlier populations stretch to Louisiana and Missouri.

The flat in Cucumber Gap was once home to a Smoky Mountains pioneer family. Look for leveled locations and piled stones in the woods, recalling forsaken lifeways. Pass some fairly large beech trees and arrow-straight regal tulip trees before descending to cross Tulip Branch at 4.4 miles. Meet the wide Jakes Creek Trail at 4.6 miles. Turn right here and descend to a pole gate at 5 miles. Enter the former summer home community, passing the Jakes Creek trailhead parking area. Keep downhill on an asphalt path (open to vehicular traffic) to a split in the road at mile 5.5. Turn right here and soon reach the Little River Trail, completing your loop at 5.6 miles.

Nearby Attractions

Elkmont has a well-kept and well-loved campground that stretches out just below the trailhead. It offers more than 200 sites.

Directions

From the junction of US 321 and US 441/Parkway in Gatlinburg (signed traffic light #3), head south on US 441 into the park. In 2.7 miles, with the Sugarlands Visitor Center on your right, turn right on Fighting Creek Gap Road and follow it south and west for 4.9 miles. Turn left on Elkmont Road at the intersection and follow it 1.3 miles to Elkmont Campground. Take the first left, just before the campground check-in station, and follow this road 0.5 mile to cross the Little River. The Little River Trail starts on the left, shortly after the bridge.

34 # Smoky Mountains:
Hen Wallow Falls

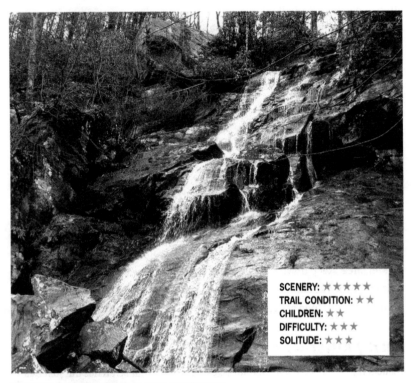

HEN WALLOW FALLS TUMBLES OVER SHEER ROCK.

GPS TRAILHEAD COORDINATES: N35° 45.470' W83° 12.578'

DISTANCE & CONFIGURATION: 4.8-mile out-and-back

HIKING TIME: 2.8 hours

HIGHLIGHTS: Tall waterfall, homesites, mountain streams

ELEVATION: 2,177' at trailhead, 3,005' at high point

ACCESS: No fees, permits, or passes required; open year-round, 24/7

MAPS: nps.gov/grsm/planyourvisit/maps.htm, USGS *Hartford*

FACILITIES: Picnic area, water fountains, restrooms, campground

WHEELCHAIR ACCESS: None

COMMENTS: No pets allowed in national park

CONTACTS: Great Smoky Mountains National Park, 865-436-1200, nps.gov/grsm

Overview

This hike leaves the Cosby area of the Smokies and travels along several tributaries of Cosby Creek, passing old homesites as it leaves flatter ground for Gabes Mountain. It continues a more-up-than-not trek deeper into the Smokies to reach Bear Neck Gap. The terrain steepens, creating ideal conditions for a precipitous waterfall. Take a spur trail to Hen Wallow Falls, a ribbon of white flowing over a rock face; crashing into a pile of rock; creating a fine, lesser-visited Smokies destination.

Route Details

Hen Wallow Falls is a lesser-visited yet scenically rewarding Smoky Mountains waterfall destinations. True, it doesn't have the volume and power of Abrams Falls, the remoteness of Ramsey Cascades, or the easy access of Indian Creek Falls. But neither does it have the crowds that flock to those cataracts. Rather, Hen Wallow Falls tumbles over a rock face, waiting for visitors. That being said, it has been a destination as long as the area has been a national park. Back in the 1930s, the Civilian Conservation Corps (CCC) routed a trail from nearby Cosby to the falls, over Gabes Mountain, passing through old-growth forest and on to Maddron Creek and the Maddron Bald Trail. The CCC trail has been rerouted somewhat, but Hen Wallow Falls still waits for visitors.

Gabes Mountain Trail begins just downhill from the entrance to the Cosby picnic area. Consider bringing a meal to enjoy here. Cosby also has a large and lesser-used campground that can serve as a fine base camp for the many trails that emanate from the area. Join a rocky track once used by mountain settlers before Great Smoky Mountains National Park came to be. Cosby was one of the most heavily settled areas in the Smokies. A pine, oak, and hickory forest shades the trail, bordered by rhododendron and mountain laurel. At 0.1 mile an old road curves left. Stay straight and gently climb to come alongside Rock Creek. True to its name, the stream tumbles noisily down a stony bed. Look down the stream to view smaller warm-up cascades. The trail continues ascending alongside Rock Creek to reach a junction at 0.3 mile. Here, a spur trail leads left 0.3 mile to Cosby Campground, allowing campers to access Gabes Mountain Trail directly. Stay right to bridge Rock Creek on a log with a handrail. The bridge allows for unobscured views of the mountain freshet.

The trail narrows as you undulate through rocky woods, stepping over streamlets flowing from Snake Den Mountain. More substantial tributaries

Smoky Mountains: Hen Wallow Falls

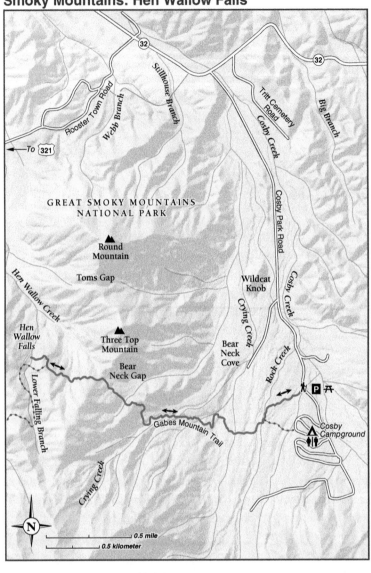

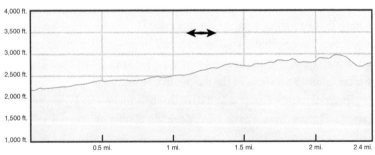

have small bridges. Black birch and rhododendron grow streamside. Ferns find their place, and moss grows on anything not moving. Bridge Crying Creek before coming to an old auto turnaround at 1.1 miles. Pick up a now-narrower trail indicated by a sign, and then climb to an old homestead—look for rocks piled in an attempt to make this hardscrabble, sloped land more arable. Continue upstream along Crying Creek before turning away at 1.3 miles to shortly pass through an unnamed gap. A little trail leads right from the gap a short distance to a lonesome grave, that of Sally Sutton, a Cosby resident. It is marked simply with a small marble marker and two stones. Dip to a small stream before rising to reach Bear Neck Gap at 1.7 miles. Rhododendron grows thick on this north-facing spot. The mountain slope sharpens considerably. Vines are draped among the trees of a cove hardwood forest. Pass an open rock face at 2 miles. In wet times water trickles down the face. Winter views of Three Top and Round Mountains open to the north. More rock bluffs lie ahead.

At 2.2 miles, reach a trail junction. Take the narrow, rooty track that leaves right toward Hen Wallow Falls. Hug a rock face on your descent, and shortly you will hear the falls. Reach the cataract at 2.4 miles. A profusion of rocks lies at the base of the 60-or-so-foot falls, which slides in a thin veil over a stone face before splattering into the boulder jumble. Since Lower Falling Branch—the stream that forms the falls—is a low-flow watercourse, consider coming here during winter or spring or after heavy rains. Don't bother with the falls you hear below. The off-trail hiking risk isn't worth the reward. If you want to explore more, continue on Gabes Mountain Trail to see another cascade upstream on Lower Falling Branch and old-growth buckeyes, silverbells, and tulip trees beyond.

Nearby Attractions

Cosby offers a fine campground and trails aplenty for the Smokies enthusiast.

Directions

From the junction of US 321 and US 441/Parkway in Gatlinburg (signed traffic light #3), head east 18.1 miles on US 321 until it comes to a T-intersection with TN 32. Follow TN 32 a little more than a mile, turning right (south) into the signed Cosby section of the park. After driving 1.9 miles up Cosby Entrance Road, watch for a road splitting left to the picnic area. Turn left here and immediately park. The Gabes Mountain Trail starts a short distance downhill, back toward the entrance to Cosby, on the west side of Cosby Entrance Road.

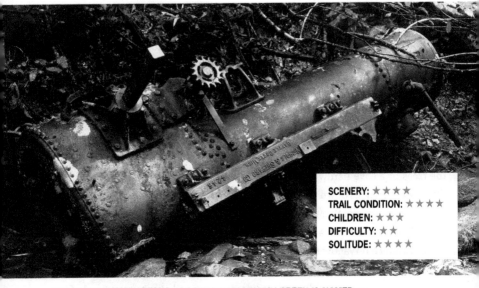

SCENERY: ★ ★ ★ ★
TRAIL CONDITION: ★ ★ ★ ★
CHILDREN: ★ ★ ★
DIFFICULTY: ★ ★
SOLITUDE: ★ ★ ★ ★

PART OF THE OLD STEAM ENGINE FOR WHICH INJUN CREEK IS NAMED

GPS TRAILHEAD COORDINATES: N35° 42.510' W83° 22.936'

DISTANCE & CONFIGURATION: 6.6-mile out-and-back

HIKING TIME: 3.8 hours

HIGHLIGHTS: Pioneer relics, solitude, old steam engine

ELEVATION: 1,680' at trailhead, 2,580' at highest point

ACCESS: No fees, permits, or passes required; open year-round, 24/7

MAPS: nps.gov/grsm/planyourvisit/maps.htm, USGS *Mount Le Conte*

FACILITIES: Restrooms, picnic area nearby

WHEELCHAIR ACCESS: None

CONTACTS: Great Smoky Mountains National Park, 865-436-1200, nps.gov/grsm

Overview

Take a walk through time on this secluded hike, which skirts the lower reaches of Mount Le Conte, passing a collection of former farms and homesites that dot the Greenbrier area of the Smokies. This underrated and underutilized Smokies trek ends at Injun Creek backcountry campsite #32, just above which lies a wrecked steam engine tractor, a high-tech contraption during the prepark days when it crashed.

Route Details

Greenbrier was one of the most heavily settled areas of what was to become Great Smoky Mountains National Park. Located in the shadow of Mount Le Conte, the rocky, mountainous area drains slopes that flow north toward Gatlinburg and Pittman Center. The land is hardly arable, but mountain settlers managed to scrape out a living along the creek bottoms and more sloped tributaries. This hike travels past several homesites located along Rhododendron Creek, a pleasant stream with which you will become very familiar during the several creek crossings the trail makes on its way up to James Gap. From there you descend into the Injun Creek watershed. The old farm–turned–backcountry campsite where you end the trek makes for a great picnic spot. Pull up a rock under the shade of a tree, or simply sprawl out on the grass and contemplate what it might have been like to live here full time without the technological accoutrements that pervade our modern life.

Start the Grapeyard Ridge Trail on a Civilian Conservation Corps–built path that cobbles together old roads used by settlers, passing rock walls and other wagon tracks splintering off the one you're following. At 0.3 mile, on a left-turning switchback, a spur path leads right to a pioneer cemetery. Sweet-gum, holly, maple, and pine form the forest. Ascend to a gap, on which sits an old homesite and the remains of a chimney, at 0.6 mile. The dull roar of the Middle Prong Little Pigeon River fades. The trail follows a small rill leading to Rhododendron Creek in a young spindly forest that was open land fourscore past. At 0.8 mile, step over the small rill and enter a persistent field. Make the first of several crossings of Rhododendron Creek and its tributaries, none of which are deep, though your shoes may get a bit wet in winter or after heavy rains.

Wind up the creek valley, noting homesites on both sides of the path. Watch for exposed trailside white quartz. The 1931 topographic map of the Smokies, commissioned by the Department of the Interior, shows 11 homes in the Rhododendron Creek watershed. Watch for more persistent fields in stream bottoms, which contrast greatly with the numerous rhododendron tunnels through which you pass. At 1.8 miles, a rock marks a spur trail leading left to a confusing network of old roads leading to forgotten homesites and graves of settlers who left the Smokies after it became a park. On down the trail, see where stones line the creek, marking a pioneer's attempt to tame Rhododendron Creek. Farmers knew this rocky land couldn't afford to lose precious topsoil to sporadic flash floods that crashed through the valley.

Smoky Mountains: Injun Creek

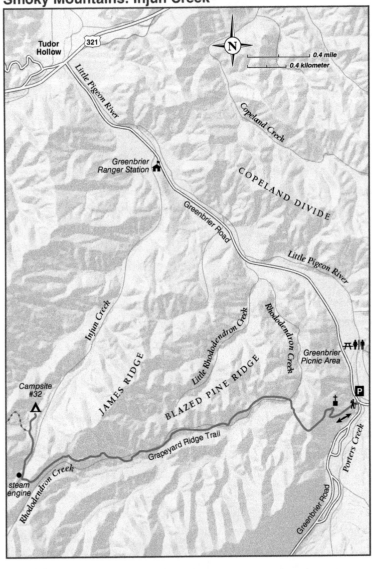

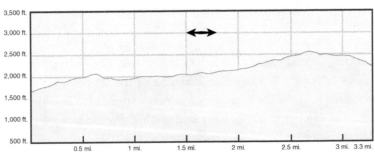

At 2.1 miles, leave Rhododendron Creek and begin the steady ascent to James Gap. A green cornucopia of rhododendron, mountain laurel, moss, and galax flank the path. Oaks and hickories stand overhead and drop their mast on the trail in fall. Another homesite, marked with a mere pile of rock rubble, sits in the saddle of James Gap at 2.8 miles. Enter the Injun Creek watershed. As you descend, the inspiration for the name Injun Creek appears in a rivulet on your right. The body and wheels of a tractorlike steam engine stand upturned, water running beneath them. Somewhere in the naming of this creek, an errant mapmaker thought the name Injun Creek referred to the Cherokee that roamed this land long ago and not a steam engine that made its final turn in the Smoky Mountains.

The old road-turned-trail descends to reach the side trail to Injun Creek backcountry campsite #32. Turn right on the side trail to the camp at 3.2 miles and enter yet another homesite. Walk around and look at the lasting changes the settlers made to the land, such as leveling the ground with rock walls. The campsite makes for a good break spot and camping spot; reserve it at smokies permits.nps.gov. On your return journey, visualize how this area will look in the future as the forest continues reestablishing its dominion over the Smokies.

Nearby Attractions

The Greenbrier area of the park offers other hiking trails, along with fishing, swimming, and picnicking.

Directions

From the junction of US 321 and US 441/Parkway in Gatlinburg (signed traffic light #3), go east on US 321/East Parkway for 6.1 miles to the Greenbrier section of the park. Turn right and drive up Greenbrier Road 3.1 miles to the intersection with Ramsey Prong Road, which crosses a bridge to your left. Park just before the intersection. The Grapeyard Ridge Trail starts on the right side of Greenbrier Road.

36 Smoky Mountains:
Little Bottoms Loop

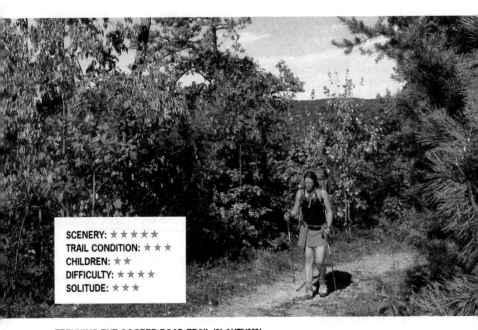

SCENERY: ★ ★ ★ ★ ★
TRAIL CONDITION: ★ ★ ★
CHILDREN: ★ ★
DIFFICULTY: ★ ★ ★ ★
SOLITUDE: ★ ★ ★

TREKKING THE COOPER ROAD TRAIL IN AUTUMN

GPS TRAILHEAD COORDINATES: N35° 36.556' W83° 56.115'

DISTANCE & CONFIGURATION: 11.3-mile balloon

HIKING TIME: 6 hours

HIGHLIGHTS: Views, Abrams Creek gorge

ELEVATION: 1,100' at trailhead, 2,050' at high point

ACCESS: No fees, permits, or passes required; open year-round, 24/7

MAPS: nps.gov/grsm/planyourvisit/maps.htm, USGS *Calderwood* and *Blockhouse*

FACILITIES: Seasonal restrooms, water fountain at Abrams Creek Campground

WHEELCHAIR ACCESS: None

CONTACTS: Great Smoky Mountains National Park, 865-436-1200, nps.gov/grsm

Overview

This long loop takes place in the Smokies' lesser-visited western lowlands. Leave Abrams Creek Ranger Station on the rolling Cooper Road Trail, passing quiet streams and fire-affected pine–oak woodlands. Join slender Hatcher Mountain

Trail to reach the Abrams Creek gorge. Travel past open rock bluffs with views, then hike beside this gorgeous stream, the Smokies' lowest-elevation waterway.

Route Details

This loop hike is easier than the mileage may indicate. It is every bit of 11.3 miles, and it's in the Smokies, but the elevation changes are neither long nor drastic. Allow ample time for rest breaks and you can make this a magnificent all-day outing. It is best hiked in fall, when the leaves are changing, but spring and winter are great too. The trail doesn't rise much above 2,000 feet, keeping winter temperatures moderate for the Smokies, and in May, blooming mountain laurels in the Abrams Creek gorge are a remarkable sight.

Leave the parking area and walk the gravel road upstream along Abrams Creek to reach the end of 16-site Abrams Creek Campground at 0.4 mile. Pass around a pole gate, joining Cooper Road Trail as it traverses a streamside flat with towering white pines overhead. Beech, maple, and holly populate the understory. Rise over a small bluff, then descend to Kingfisher Branch at 0.9 mile. The trail and stream become one for a short distance, then divide.

Reach a trail junction at 1.3 miles. Your return route, Little Bottoms Trail, leaves right. Keep straight on Cooper Road Trail, shortly passing Cooper Road backcountry campsite #1. This former homesite is the lowest-elevation backcountry campsite in the park. It's odd to contemplate, but the rich woods through which you travel were a farmer's cornfield a century back. Continue upstream, stepping over Kingfisher Creek at 1.9 miles. Hike uphill more than not in a white pine–white oak complex. Step over a tributary of Buck Shank Branch at 2.7 miles. Level off in Gold Mine Gap at 3 miles. Stay with Cooper Road Trail as it descends steeply and then levels off to reach another trail junction at 3.4 miles. Here, Cane Creek Trail keeps straight, but Cooper Road Trail, our route, curves right and uphill past Rugel's Rocks, so named for the two massive boulders that block the path, effectively keeping vehicles from continuing, as they did in early park days. Cooper Road, named for the foreman who built it, was used to connect Cades Cove to the Chilhowee area.

Level off at 4 miles, entering a recovering burn. The scraggly forest may not look so pretty, but periodic fire is necessary to maintain the ecosystem. The fires have also opened more views of Chilhowee Mountain and the tower of Look Rock to the northwest and other ridges to the south. The sandy, gravelly track undulates through more low woods with views, then reaches a four-way

Smoky Mountains: Little Bottoms Loop

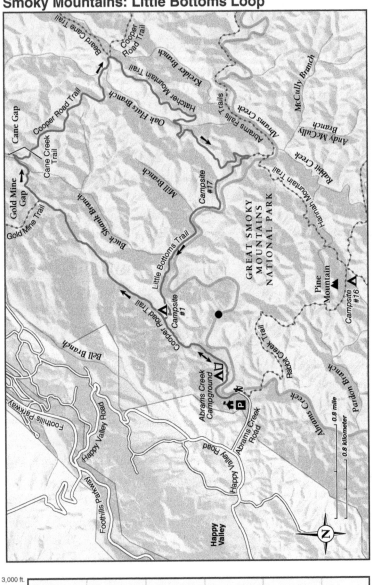

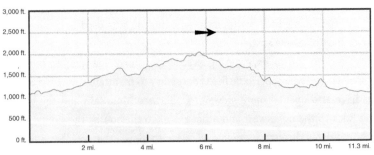

trail junction at 5.3 miles. Turn right here, southbound, joining the singletrack Hatcher Mountain Trail. Westerly views open through the pines, maples, and gum trees rising above blueberry bushes. Slip from the east side to the west side of the mountain at 5.7 miles, now going downhill more than not.

At 6.6 miles, step over Oak Flats Branch in a rhododendron thicket. Soon cross a tributary. Return to dry woods, curving into declivitous Abrams Creek gorge at 7.4 miles. On a clear winter day, Gregory Bald is visible from here. Dip to a hollow full of dwarf irises, then meet Little Bottoms Trail at 7.8 miles. Turn right here, westbound, entering the Abrams Creek gorge. It isn't long before you pass through open rock bluffs bordered by fire-scarred woods. Views open of Look Rock Tower and Chilhowee Mountain, which separates the Smokies from greater Knoxville. The rugged hiker-only path, nicknamed the Goat Trail, dips to reach the spur trail to Little Bottoms backcountry campsite #17 at 8.4 miles, then saddles alongside Abrams Creek. Enjoy close-up stream panoramas while occasionally climbing mountain laurel–cloaked hillsides. Step over Buck Shank Branch at 9.4 miles, then surmount a low ridge. Cruise through young forest. A pair of switchbacks drops you into thick forest along Kingfisher Creek, and you'll encounter a trail junction at 10 miles. You have now completed the loop portion of the hike. It's an easy 1.3-mile backtrack to the Abrams Creek parking area.

Nearby Attractions

Abrams Creek has an intimate and attractive 16-site primitive campground generally open from March through October. For exact dates, visit nps.gov/grsm.

Directions

From the intersection of US 411/TN 33 and US 129/TN 115 in Maryville, take US 129 (Alcoa Highway) south for 7 miles. At the four-way intersection, bear right to continue south on US 129. In 3.6 miles, bear left at the T to keep south on US 129, and continue 7.1 miles to Chilhowee Lake. Just past the intersection with the Foothills Parkway, turn left (north) on Happy Valley Road, following it 5.9 miles to Abrams Creek Road. Turn right on Abrams Creek Road and drive 0.7 mile, passing the ranger station. The parking area is on the right just after the ranger station. The Cooper Road Trail starts at the rear of Abrams Creek Campground. Park your car in the designated area near the ranger station. *Do not park in the campground, which is gated during the cold season.*

Smoky Mountains: Porters Flat

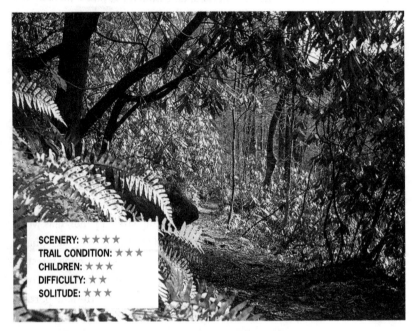

SCENERY: ★ ★ ★ ★
TRAIL CONDITION: ★ ★ ★
CHILDREN: ★ ★ ★
DIFFICULTY: ★ ★
SOLITUDE: ★ ★ ★

THE SMOKY MOUNTAINS DESERVE THEIR NATIONAL PARK STATUS.

GPS TRAILHEAD COORDINATES: N35° 41.814' W83° 23.272'

DISTANCE & CONFIGURATION: 3.6-mile out-and-back

HIKING TIME: 2 hours

HIGHLIGHTS: Waterfall, preserved hemlock grove, homestead

ELEVATION: 1,950' at trailhead, 2,510' at turnaround point

ACCESS: No fees, permits, or passes required; open year-round, 24/7

MAPS: nps.gov/grsm/planyourvisit/maps.htm, USGS *Mount Le Conte*

FACILITIES: Restrooms, picnic area nearby

WHEELCHAIR ACCESS: None

COMMENTS: Porters Creek Valley is one of the Smokies' most bountiful wildflower destinations, so consider hiking here during spring.

CONTACTS: Great Smoky Mountains National Park, 865-436-1200, nps.gov/grsm

Overview

This trek in the Greenbrier area of the Smokies travels along a crystalline mountain stream to reach a preserved hemlock grove. Next, you hike to a delicate falls streaming over a rock face. On your outgoing or return trip, stop by a former farmstead, complete with historic wood structures.

Route Details

This hike offers many highlights that will have you stopping and enjoying them, unable to get up a head of steam if you are hiking purely for exercise. The valley of Porters Creek, through which you will travel, was heavily populated before the Smokies became a park. Even today, hikers will see squared-off flats, stone steps, and more. This hike visits the Ownby Cemetery as well as the Messer place, a homesite that was early headquarters for the Smoky Mountains Hiking Club. Also, you will view a hemlock grove being preserved by the park. The dark-green cathedral stands out among today's saddening skeletal remains of most hemlock trees. Finally, travel farther up Porters Creek to a cascade known as Fern Branch Falls. The slender, low-flow stream spills over a tall rock slab but will nearly dry in late summer and fall.

Leave the trailhead, passing around a pole gate on a wide gravel track. Straight-trunked tulip trees rise among doghobble, rhododendron, and ferns. Black birch and buckeye thrive in this boulder-strewn area astride Porters Creek. The translucent waters of the braided mountain stream reveal gray and pale rocks. The walking is easy. Potato Ridge rises steeply to your right. Begin looking for pioneer relics. In winter you will more easily see the old rock walls and stone steps—the remains of an East Tennessee way of life long abandoned—such as that seen at 0.6 mile on your right.

Bridge Long Branch at 0.7 mile. Just ahead, the Ownby Cemetery is on your right. You are officially in Porters Flat, a relatively level area surrounded by steep ridges. Pass metal parts of an abandoned jalopy before reaching an old auto turnaround and the preserved hemlock grove. The deep, dark greenery was once a common sight in the Smokies, but the hemlock woolly adelgid has devastated the park's estimated 137,000 acres of hemlock woodlands, though conservation areas like this one are being preserved by spraying for the pest, soil drenching with insecticide, and releasing beetles that attack the adelgid.

Two trails spur from the hemlock-shaded auto turnaround. Here, Brushy Mountain Trail leads west to Trillium Gap on the shoulder of Mount Le Conte, and an unnamed but signed spur trail leads right 200 yards to the old Messer Farmstead. Go ahead and visit the homesite, taking a wide path that curves to a clearing centered around a cantilever barn, a popular style of barn in the prepark

Smoky Mountains: Porters Flat

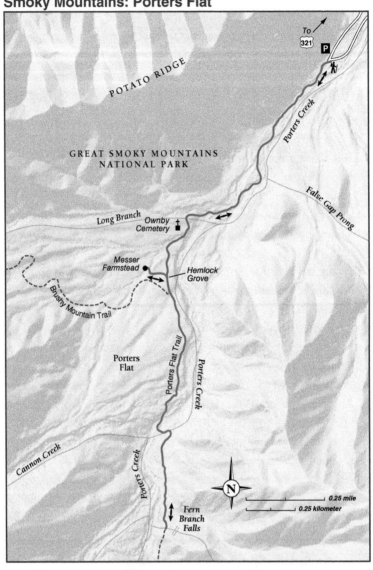

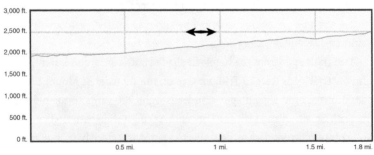

Smokies. Two log cribs hold up the overhanging larger portion. The structure is not entirely original; its wood-shingle roof has been replaced along with other elements as needed. Just ahead is the springhouse. Then you reach a homestead occupied by several different owners, the last one being John Messer. These structures were reconfigured into the Smoky Mountains Hiking Club building we see today. Note the low roof and rock fireplaces.

Resume your hike up the now-narrower Porters Flat Trail. Mossy boulders and ferns line the natural-surface track. Bridge Porters Creek at 1.5 miles. Take advantage of this view to absorb the stream scenery, where huge boulders form impediments to frothing water determined to leave its high-country point of origin for Middle Prong Little Pigeon River below.

During spring you have already seen many a wildflower, but beyond here the colorful signs of rebirth reach their densest concentrations. The forest floor is colored with white, purple, yellow, and pink. Old-growth buckeye, white oak, and Carolina silverbell rise among the flower fields. The path narrows and steepens as the northern edge of Porters Mountain rises to your left on the mountainside. In summer stinging nettle will brush against unprotected legs.

At 1.8 miles, look left as slender Fern Branch Falls splashes over an open rock slab to your left. You're more likely to hear it before you see it. The unnamed stream of the falls trickles over the trail. A boulder field stands between you and the cataract, but the falls are easily visible from the trail and make a fitting turn-around point to a great hike. In winter, spring, or after heavy rains, the ribbon of white will be more dramatic. If you want to extend your hike, continue 1.4 miles farther to Porters Flat backcountry campsite #31, where the trail dead-ends. Either way, be sure to look for more pioneer evidence on your return trip.

Nearby Attractions

The Greenbrier area of the park offers other hiking trails, along with fishing, swimming, and picnicking.

Directions

From signed traffic light #3 on US 441 in Gatlinburg, take US 321/East Parkway 6.1 miles to the Greenbrier section of the park. Turn right, drive up Greenbrier Road 4 miles, and park at the end of the dead-end loop.

38   Smoky Mountains:
Rich Mountain Loop

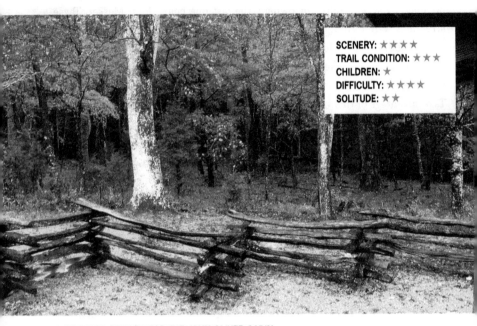

A SPLIT-RAIL FENCE NEAR THE JOHN OLIVER CABIN

GPS TRAILHEAD COORDINATES: N35° 36.400' W83° 46.655'

DISTANCE & CONFIGURATION: 8.5-mile loop

HIKING TIME: 4.8 hours

HIGHLIGHTS: John Oliver Cabin, multiple views

ELEVATION: 1,940' at trailhead, 3,686' at high point

ACCESS: No fees, permits, or passes required; open year-round, 24/7

MAPS: nps.gov/grsm/planyourvisit/maps.htm, USGS *Cades Cove* and *Kinzel Springs*

FACILITIES: Picnic area, campground, water, camp store (seasonal) nearby

WHEELCHAIR ACCESS: None

CONTACTS: Great Smoky Mountains National Park, 865-436-1200, nps.gov/grsm

Overview

This excellent Smokies day hike shows Cades Cove from a different perspective, a top-down look at the historic farming community nestled against the crest of the mountains. Stop by the historic cabin of Cades Cove resident John Oliver, adding a tangible touch to this exploration of the human and natural history of Knoxville's nearby national park.

Route Details

This is perhaps the quintessential Smoky Mountains loop hike. It starts in Cades Cove, a point of pride for the Volunteer State, then wanders west along the foot of Rich Mountain, tracing pioneer roads with views of Cades Cove. When the John Oliver Cabin appears at the wood's edge, you'll walk through pioneer history. Then the jaunt morphs into an ascent of Rich Mountain. Here, you travel along a ridgetop and the park border, gaining southerly views of the dark, wooded state-line ridge across Cades Cove and northerly views into Tuckaleechee Cove. Visit the former mountaintop tower site at Cerulean Knob, then mostly descend a winding, gravelly track with enough switchbacks to make you dizzy.

Start your hike on Rich Mountain Loop Trail, a singletrack dirt-and-rock path. Cades Cove Loop Road is to your left, and Crooked Arm Ridge rises to your right. The nearly level path is shaded by white pines, oaks, and tulip trees. By 0.3 mile, fields open to your left. Gain bucolic views through the trees of waving grasses with wooded mountains beyond. At 0.5 mile, rock-hop over seasonal Crooked Arm Branch, then come to a trail junction. Here, Crooked Arm Ridge Trail, your return route, leaves right. Stay straight with Rich Mountain Loop Trail as it moseys through slightly hilly, wooded terrain heavy with shortleaf pines, indicating this was likely pasture or cropland in Cades Cove's heyday a century back. Cross a small rocky branch at 0.8 mile as you keep a rolling westerly course amid more pines and sourwood. At 1 mile, step over Harrison Branch. Wander more foothills, then emerge into a clearing at the John Oliver Cabin at 1.4 miles. Built in 1820, the cabin serves as a link to East Tennessee's rural past. Oliver was an early settler of the cove and helped populate it with his many offspring. Other visitors access the cabin from Cades Cove Loop Road.

Leave the cabin and abruptly turn right, up Marthas Branch, northbound on sloping, stony land. Note the older trees directly beside the road-turned-trail. The hollow narrows and you pass a crumbled chimney on your right at 1.6 miles. Cross Marthas Branch at 1.7 miles. The trail steepens. At 1.9 miles, the path clambers over an open rock slab. Notice the scratch marks from horseshoes scraping over the rock. At 2 miles, step over Marthas Branch again. Leave the stream for good at 2.2 miles, and begin arcing around Cave Ridge amidst pine and black gum trees. Big boulders appear in the forest. At 2.9 miles, on a switchback, glance

Smoky Mountains: Rich Mountain Loop

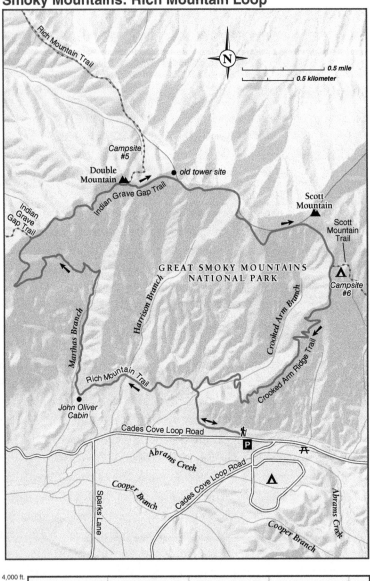

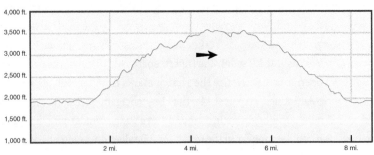

down at Cades Cove—the fields seem a lot smaller! You are now at 3,000 feet. At 3.3 miles, meet Indian Grave Gap Trail on the ridgecrest of Rich Mountain.

Join Indian Grave Gap Trail as it gently climbs along Rich Mountain. Gain obscured views across Cades Cove. At 4.2 miles, Rich Mountain Trail leaves left. Backcountry campsite #5 is just down that path. Continue up Indian Grave Gap Trail and enjoy the opening views. Reach a junction at 4.4 miles. Here, a spur trail leads left to the old fire tower atop Cerulean Knob. The four concrete tower supports remain, as does a flat below the knob, with a well or catch basin to serve the tower keeper's cabin once located there. The forest cover limits the views now, but the clearing makes an ideal picnic spot.

Start descending easily along Rich Mountain. Enjoy your hard-earned highland forest cruise. More northerly views open into Tuckaleechee Cove. Pass an odd flat (once a power-line pad) before meeting Scott Mountain Trail at 5.8 miles. Stay right, joining Crooked Arm Ridge Trail. The path soon divides, then comes back together in a brief confusing section. Switchback down toward Cades Cove. One turn follows another on the rocky path. Some trail users have shortcut the switchbacks. Don't follow their lead, as erosion follows shortcuts.

Step over Crooked Arm Branch at 7.6 miles. Trace the stream downhill on a moderate slope and intersect Rich Mountain Loop Trail at 8 miles. From here, backtrack to reach the trailhead at 8.5 miles.

Nearby Attractions

Bicyclers love the 10-mile **Cades Cove Loop Road.** The road is closed to vehicles Wednesday and Saturday mornings before 10 a.m. during the warm season, but bicyclists can pedal it anytime from dawn to dusk, although auto traffic can make the ride less inviting.

Directions

From Knoxville, take US 129 South (Alcoa Highway) south to Maryville; then join US 321 South toward Smoky Mountains National Park. In Townsend, where US 321 goes left at a traffic light, stay straight, joining TN 73 to reach the park entrance in 1.4 miles. Head forward to the Townsend Wye, a split in the road, in 0.9 mile. Turn right here, onto Laurel Creek Road, and follow it 7.4 miles to the beginning of Cades Cove Loop Road. Park at the loop's beginning in the large parking area on the left. To pick up Rich Mountain Loop Trail, walk a short distance down the loop road, past the pole gate; the signed trails begin on your right.

39 Smoky Mountains: Walker Sisters'
Place via Little Greenbrier Trail

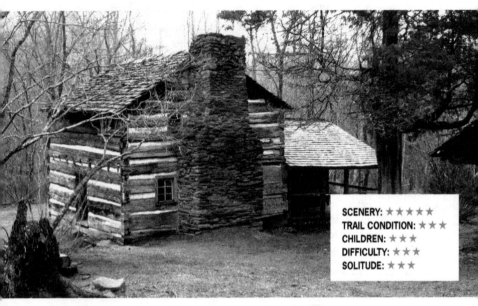

SCENERY: ★ ★ ★ ★ ★
TRAIL CONDITION: ★ ★ ★
CHILDREN: ★ ★ ★
DIFFICULTY: ★ ★ ★
SOLITUDE: ★ ★ ★

THE FORMER CABIN OF THE WALKER SISTERS, WHO WERE AMONG THE LAST NATIVE SMOKY MOUNTAIN RESIDENTS

GPS TRAILHEAD COORDINATES: N35° 41.678' W83° 38.759'

DISTANCE & CONFIGURATION: 5-mile out-and-back

HIKING TIME: 3 hours

HIGHLIGHTS: Mountain views, historic Smoky Mountain homestead

ELEVATION: 1,890' at trailhead, 2,280' at high point

ACCESS: No fees, permits, or passes required; open year-round, 24/7

MAPS: nps.gov/grsm/planyourvisit/maps.htm, USGS *Wear Cove*

FACILITIES: None

WHEELCHAIR ACCESS: None

COMMENTS: No pets allowed in national park

CONTACTS: Great Smoky Mountains National Park, 865-436-1200, nps.gov/grsm

Overview

This scenic ridgeline hike presents views, then visits one of the last working pioneer homesteads in the Smokies. Start at a gap on the Little Greenbrier Trail straddling the national park boundary. The vistas are numerous from a pine-cloaked mountainside before you reach a second gap. Descend a hollow and reach the Walker Sisters' place, occupied by the siblings until 1964.

Route Details

This hike travels a ridgeline that seemingly divides time periods in East Tennessee. On one side, there is the preserved Smoky Mountains National Park, where the Walker Sisters' cabin—your destination—exemplifies a simpler time, when the Smokies were truly the back of beyond, where homesteaders would spend a lifetime and maybe never even get to Knoxville, much less more distant places. On the other side of the ridge, we see modern homesteaders staking out a home in Wears Valley to be near the beauty that is the national park, changing it from a land of the forgotten to an urban outpost. Your mind may contemplate such things as you walk the ridge, known as Little Mountain, that forms the border of the Smokies.

Begin the hike at Wear Cove Gap on the Little Greenbrier Trail. Climb through archetypal pine–oak–mountain laurel forest on a narrow pathway. Blueberries are abundant in sunnier locales. The path skirts the park border in several places—you will see boundary signs here and there. Look down at the elaborate stonework by trail makers that keeps the path from sliding down the mountainside. Views open north beyond the park, especially at a gap at 0.5 mile.

Hike more up than down, then curve around the south side of Little Mountain at 1 mile. Listen for flowing water in the lowlands below. Enjoy good looks into the heart of the park. The walking is easy, allowing you to enjoy more views of Wear Cove and Cove Mountain to the east. Descend the ridge of Little Mountain to reach Little Brier Gap and a trail junction at mile 1.9. Turn right here, joining Little Brier Gap Trail, descending into the moist cove of Little Brier Branch, flowing to your left. Tulip trees join the forest.

The V-shaped hollow widens. Little Brier Branch gains flow from tributaries. Reach a signed trail junction at 2.3 miles. Little Brier Gap Trail keeps forward as a gravel road, while a spur track leads left to the Walker Sisters' place. Turn left along tiny Straight Cove Branch. The preponderance of tulip trees and shortleaf pines indicates the area was once cleared. Imagine these trailside flats as fields of corn and other vegetables, perhaps some pasture, back when this was an active homestead.

Smoky Mountains:
Walker Sisters' Place via Little Greenbrier Trail

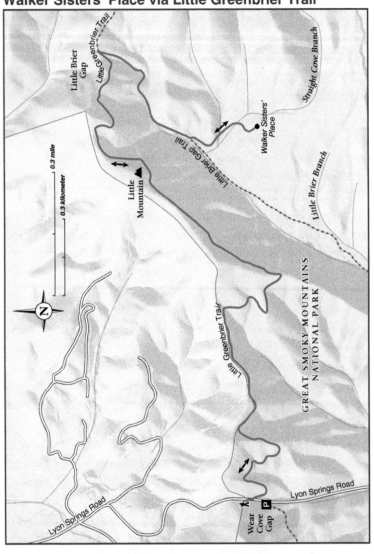

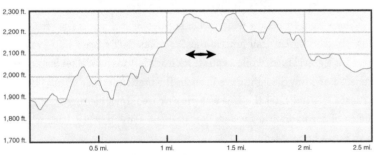

Come to an open area at 2.5 miles and reach the Walker Sisters' place in a grassy clearing. This cove was occupied for 150 years, with the Walker sisters remaining after the national park was established, thanks to a lifetime lease agreement. After they passed away, the park preserved their homestead. Now, the springhouse, main home, and small barn remain. Notice the notched-log construction of the buildings and the nonnative ornamental bushes. Walk inside— the low roof required less construction material and also made the home easier to heat. The white stuff on the walls is old pieces of newspaper that were used to brighten and insulate the cabin. A ladder leads to the sleeping loft. The large fireplace warmed the home, and heat rising up the rock chimney kept loft sleepers a little toastier. The springhouse not only kept critters from fouling the water but also helped keep milk and butter cool in the summertime. The barn is a smaller version of the cantilever-type barn popular in East Tennessee a century and more ago. Note the farm implements on the wall. If you walk around the perimeter of the yard, you will see other relics, including old car tires that the Walker sisters likely regarded as junk. Remember to leave all artifacts so others can enjoy and discover them. If you are further interested in the area's history, continue down Little Brier Gap Trail 1.1 more miles to the Little Greenbrier Schoolhouse before returning to Wear Cove Gap.

Nearby Attractions

Metcalf Bottoms is 1.3 miles from Wear Cove Gap into the Smokies. It offers picnicking and restrooms alongside Little River.

Directions

From Knoxville, take US 129 South (Alcoa Highway) south to Maryville; then join US 321 South toward Smoky Mountains National Park. In Townsend, where US 321 goes left at a traffic light, stay straight, joining TN 73 to reach the park entrance at Townsend in 1.4 miles. Head forward to reach the Townsend Wye, a split in the road, in 0.9 mile. Turn left here, onto Little River Road, and follow it 7.8 miles to the Metcalf Bottoms Picnic Area. Turn left into Metcalf Bottoms Picnic Area, crossing the Little River on a bridge. Continue on the road 1.3 miles to the park border, where the Little Greenbrier Trail starts on the right. There is parking here for only one car directly by the trail; another parking area is just over the hill from the trailhead.

40 # Smoky Mountains:
Whiteoak Sink

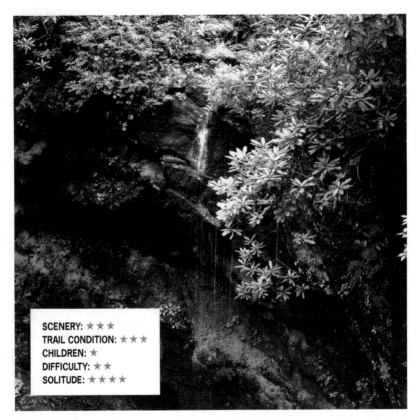

SCENERY: ★ ★ ★
TRAIL CONDITION: ★ ★ ★
CHILDREN: ★
DIFFICULTY: ★ ★
SOLITUDE: ★ ★ ★ ★

WHITEOAK SINK IS HOME TO AN INTRICATE PLUMBING SYSTEM.

GPS TRAILHEAD COORDINATES: N35° 37.633' W83° 43.588'

DISTANCE & CONFIGURATION: 4.6-mile out-and-back

HIKING TIME: 2.8 hours

HIGHLIGHTS: Cave, sinkhole, waterfall, spring wildflowers

ELEVATION: 1,650' at trailhead, 1,835' at high point

ACCESS: No fees, permits, or passes required; open year-round, 24/7

MAPS: nps.gov/grsm/planyourvisit/maps.htm, USGS *Wear Cove*

FACILITIES: None

WHEELCHAIR ACCESS: None

CONTACTS: Great Smoky Mountains National Park, 865-436-1200, nps.gov/grsm

Overview

Take a walk to an off-the-beaten-path Smokies destination—a sinkhole near Cades Cove. Follow an easy track for a little over 1 mile, then dip into Whiteoak Sink, once home to pioneer families. The sink is also home to some complicated underground plumbing. You can see this manifested in a cave, as well as in a waterfall that drops off a rock face only to disappear into a sink.

Route Details

Even though this Smoky Mountains hike encompasses some hiking on an unmarked trail, the way is clear and the path itself is maintained by the National Park Service, sort of an unadvertised trail. The park service is skittish about too many people coming here because of concerns about rare plants above ground and life in the caves down here. Don't even think about trying to head underground, for your own safety and to allow the belowground habitat to remain undisturbed. You will first follow a historic road built by the first president of nearby Maryville College, Dr. Isaac Anderson. He built the road to connect with settlements over on Hazel Creek in North Carolina, with the intention of sharing Christianity with them. The road was built only to the state line then abandoned. Residents of nearby Cades Cove used what became known as Anderson Turnpike to reach the Blount County seat in Maryville.

The hike then follows the clear unnamed trail into Whiteoak Sink. The singletrack path wanders along the slope of a streamlet before dropping off into the flats within Whiteoak Sink, a bowl-like depression encircled by hills. Streams here have no outlet and drain into the ground below. Early residents found the level sink desirable for farming, and several families resided here. Now the sink is left to the flora and fauna, highlighted by impressive spring wildflower displays.

Once in Whiteoak Sink you can visit two different highlights: First, stop by a cave backed against a rock bluff. Then, a short backtrack will take you to a deep sinkhole into which a waterfall spills, a live demonstration of the intricate underground plumbing in this part of the Smoky Mountains. Just remember to stay on the trail and give this special place the respect it deserves.

Join the wide Schoolhouse Gap Trail as it descends briefly toward Laurel Creek then turns up Spence Branch. Travel directly alongside the small clear stream as it flows over rock slabs in small stairstep cascades. The wide path is shaded by sycamores, witch hazel, and birches. Rhododendron finds its place as the trail heads up a cool, moist hollow, bridging Spence Branch at 0.1 mile. The

Smoky Mountains: Whiteoak Sink

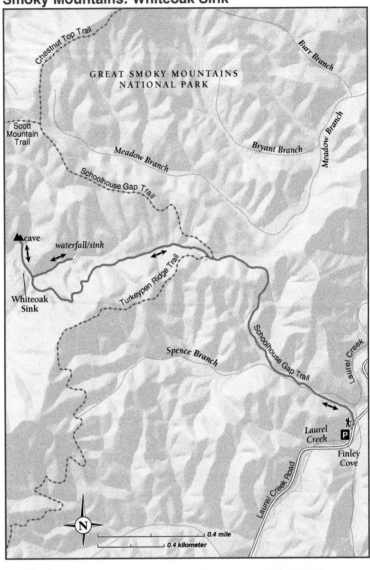

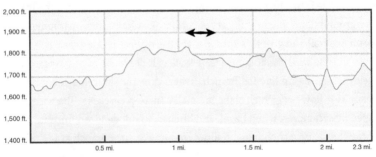

track suddenly steepens at 0.5 mile, as it heads up a tributary of Spence Branch. Level off in a gap and high point at 0.8 mile. Swing past a persistent clearing on your right. Reach Dorsey Gap and a trail junction at 1.1 miles. Here, Turkeypen Ridge Trail leaves left for Laurel Creek Road, while our hike keeps straight on Schoolhouse Gap Trail. Just ahead, on your left, is the trail to Whiteoak Sink. The path is clearly visible as it descends left. A stile fence blocks passage by horses and is your "for certain" marker that this is the way to Whiteoak Sink.

Begin working downhill in a moist valley. Despite not being on maps, the trail is maintained, as evidenced by trailside sawn logs. Come along and cross a small stream in young forest at 1.4 miles. Continue a slim path on a slope. Descend steeply to the sink, entering a flat and rich wildflower area to make a junction at 1.9 miles. Here, trails go left and right. Head left first, walking level ground from which rise regal tulip trees. The trail dead-ends at a gray cliff and cave. The cave is protected by a gate to prevent entry. Other user-created trails explore the flat.

Backtrack to the junction in Whiteoak Sink. This time take the other path, traveling east through more of the hill-guarded plain. Soon the sounds of splashing water drift into your ears, and you reach the waterfall and sink at 2.4 miles. Here, the streamlet you followed into Whiteoak Sink tumbles over a rock bluff, splashing 30 feet onto rocks and disappearing in a dark, wet maw. In winter, icicles form on the lip of the falls, adding frosty splendor. Do not walk into the sinkhole. Leave it for the permanent residents of Whiteoak Sink. Backtrack to the trailhead, making sure to stay on the established trails.

Nearby Attractions

Bicyclers love to pedal 10-mile **Cades Cove Loop Road.** It is closed to vehicles Wednesday and Saturday mornings before 10 a.m. during the warm season, but bicyclists can pedal the road anytime from dawn to dusk.

Directions

From Knoxville, take US 129 South (Alcoa Highway) south to Maryville; then join US 321 South toward Smoky Mountains National Park. In Townsend, where US 321 goes left at a traffic light, stay straight, joining TN 73 to reach the park entrance at Townsend in 1.4 miles. Head forward to reach the Townsend Wye, a split in the road, in 0.9 mile. Turn right here, onto Laurel Creek Road, and follow it 3.7 miles to the Schoolhouse Gap Trail parking area, on your right.

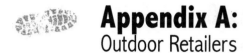

Appendix A:
Outdoor Retailers

Below is contact information for outdoor retailers in the Knoxville metro area.

BASS PRO SHOP
3629 Outdoor Sportsman Place
Sevierville, TN 37764
865-932-5600
basspro.com

RIVER SPORTS
2918 Sutherland Ave.
Knoxville, TN 37919
865-523-0066
riversportsoutfitters.com

DICKS SPORTING GOODS
221 N. Peters Road
Knoxville, TN 37923
865-531-2221
dickssportinggoods.com

UNCLE LEMS OUTFITTERS
2450 Parkway
Pigeon Forge, TN 37863
865-366-1455
unclelems.com

LITTLE RIVER TRADING COMPANY
2408 E. Lamar Alexander Parkway
Maryville, TN 37804
865-681-4141
littlerivertradingco.com

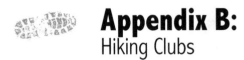 # Appendix B:
Hiking Clubs

The Knoxville metro area is home to many hiking enthusiasts. Here are some good contacts for clubs and groups that welcome your participation.

SMOKY MOUNTAIN HIKING CLUB
smhclub.org

UNIVERSITY OF TENNESSEE CANOE AND HIKING CLUB
utk.campuslabs.com/engage/organization/canoeandhiking

GREAT SMOKY MOUNTAINS HIKING AND ADVENTURE GROUP
meetup.com/great-smokies-hiking-adventure-group

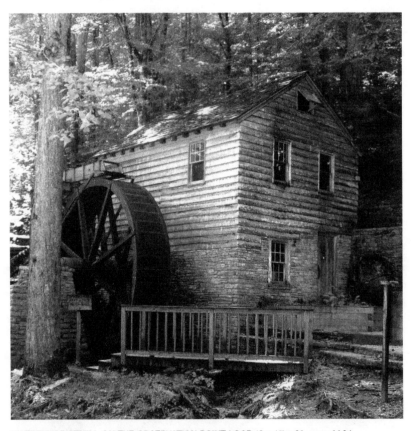

HISTORIC GRISTMILL ON THE OBSERVATION POINT LOOP *(See Hike 21, page 110.)*

Index

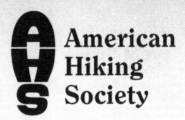

American Hiking Society

PROTECT THE PLACES YOU LOVE TO HIKE.

Become a member today and
take $5 off using the code **Hike5**.

AmericanHiking.org/join

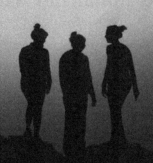

American Hiking Society is the only
national nonprofit organization dedicated
to empowering all to enjoy, share, and
preserve the hiking experience.

Check out this great title from
Wilderness Press!

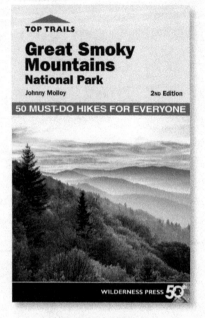

Top Trails:
Great Smoky Mountains National Park

Johnny Molloy   5 x 8, paperback
ISBN: 978-0-89997-876-5   416 pages
$18.95, 2nd Edition   maps and photos

Johnny Molloy, who has spent more than 800 nights backpacking in the Smokies, has updated his classic guide *Top Trails: Great Smoky Mountains National Park*. This revised edition has been completely updated, including the new backcountry reservation system implemented in the park.

He has also added some excellent hikes, some of them well off the beaten path. For example, the hike to Baskins Creek Falls takes you past a pioneer homesite and to a scenic cascade overshadowed by more popular waterfalls nearby, making it an ideal destination for those who want to escape the crowds.

Additionally, Johnny—who considers the Smokies his home stomping ground—makes sure that all the necessary information to help you execute a hike (from directions to maps) is correct. New photos add flair to the book.

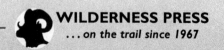

WILDERNESS PRESS
... on the trail since 1967

DEAR CUSTOMERS AND FRIENDS,

SUPPORTING YOUR INTEREST IN OUTDOOR ADVENTURE, travel, and an active lifestyle is central to our operations, from the authors we choose to the locations we detail to the way we design our books. Menasha Ridge Press was incorporated in 1982 by a group of veteran outdoorsmen and professional outfitters. For many years now, we've specialized in creating books that benefit the outdoors enthusiast.

Almost immediately, Menasha Ridge Press earned a reputation for revolutionizing outdoors- and travel-guidebook publishing. For such activities as canoeing, kayaking, hiking, backpacking, and mountain biking, we established new standards of quality that transformed the whole genre, resulting in outdoor-recreation guides of great sophistication and solid content. Menasha Ridge Press continues to be outdoor publishing's greatest innovator.

The folks at Menasha Ridge Press are as at home on a whitewater river or mountain trail as they are editing a manuscript. The books we build for you are the best they can be, because we're responding to your needs. Plus, we use and depend on them ourselves.

We look forward to seeing you on the river or the trail. If you'd like to contact us directly, visit us at menasharidge.com. We thank you for your interest in our books and the natural world around us all.

SAFE TRAVELS,

Bob Sehlinger

BOB SEHLINGER
PUBLISHER

About the Author

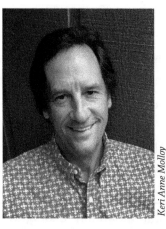

JOHNNY MOLLOY is a writer and adventurer based in East Tennessee who lived in Knoxville for 20 years. His passion for the outdoors started on a backpacking trip in Great Smoky Mountains National Park. That first foray unleashed a love of the outdoors that led to his spending countless nights backpacking, canoe camping, and tent camping over the past three decades. Friends enjoyed his outdoor adventure stories, and one even suggested he write a book. He pursued his friend's idea and soon parlayed his hobby into an occupation. His efforts have resulted in more than 75 books. His writings include hiking guidebooks, camping guidebooks, paddling guidebooks, comprehensive guidebooks about specific areas, and true outdoor adventure books. Johnny has also written numerous magazine articles for websites and newspapers. He continues writing and traveling extensively throughout the United States, endeavoring in a variety of outdoor pursuits. His nonoutdoor interests include serving Jesus as a Gideon, American history, and University of Tennessee sports. For the latest on Johnny, please visit johnnymolloy.com.

Keri Anne Molloy